KEY TOPICS IN
RESPIRATORY MEDICINE

The KEY TOPICS Series

Advisors:

T.M. Craft *Department of Anaesthesia and Intensive Care, Royal United Hospital, Bath, UK*
C.S. Garrard *Intensive Therapy Unit, John Radcliffe Hospital, Oxford, UK*
P.M. Upton *Department of Anaesthetics, Royal Cornwall Hospital, Treliske, Truro, UK*

Anaesthesia, Second Edition

Obstetrics and Gynaecology, Second Edition

Accident and Emergency Medicine

Paediatrics, Second Edition

Orthopaedic Surgery

Otolaryngology

Ophthalmology

Psychiatry

General Surgery

Renal Medicine

Trauma

Chronic Pain

Oral and Maxillofacial Surgery

Oncology

Cardiovascular Medicine

Neurology

Neonatology

Gastroenterology

Thoracic Surgery

Respiratory Medicine

Forthcoming titles include:

Orthopaedic Trauma Surgery

Critical Care

Accident and Emergency Medicine, Second Edition

KEY TOPICS IN
RESPIRATORY MEDICINE

W.J.M. KINNEAR
MD, FRCP
Consultant Physician, University Hospital,
Nottingham, UK

I.D.A. JOHNSTON
MD, FRCP
Consultant Physician, University Hospital,
Nottingham, UK

I.P. HALL
DM, FRCP
Reader in Molecular Medicine, University of Nottingham and
Honorary Consultant Physician, University Hospital,
Nottingham, UK

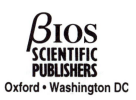

β**IOS**
SCIENTIFIC
PUBLISHERS
Oxford • Washington DC

© BIOS Scientific Publishers Limited, 1999

First published 1999

A CIP catalogue record for this book is available from the British Library.

ISBN 1 85996 271 8

BIOS Scientific Publishers Ltd
9 Newtec Place, Magdalen Road, Oxford OX4 1RE, UK
Tel. +44 (0)1865 726286. Fax. +44 (0)1865 246823
World Wide Web home page: http://www.bios.co.uk/

Important Note from the Publisher
The information contained within this book was obtained by BIOS Scientific Publishers Ltd from sources believed by us to be reliable. However, while every effort has been made to ensure its accuracy, no responsibility for loss or injury whatsoever occasioned to any person acting or refraining from action as a result of information contained herein can be accepted by the authors or publishers.

The reader should remember that medicine is a constantly evolving science and while the authors and publishers have ensured that all dosages, applications and practices are based on current indications, there may be specific practices which differ between communities. You should always follow the guidelines laid down by the manufacturers of specific products and the relevant authorities in the country in which you are practising.

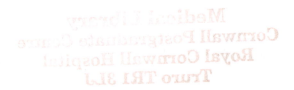
Production Editor: Andrea Bosher.
Typeset by J&L Composition Ltd, Filey, UK.
Printed by T.J. International Ltd, Padstow, UK.

CONTENTS

ABBREVIATIONS

ABPA	allergic bronchopulmonary aspergillus
ACTH	adrenocorticotrophic hormone
ANCA	anti-neutrophil cytoplasmic antibodies
anti-GBM	anti-glomerular basement membrane
AP	alveolar proteinosis
ARDS	adult respiratory distress syndrome
AVM	arterio-venous malformations
BAL	bronchoalveolar lavage
BCG	Bacille Calmette–Guérin
BHL	bilateral hilar lymphadenopathy
BOOP	bronchiolitis obliterans organizing pneumonia
BTS	British Thoracic Society
CF	cystic fibrosis
CFA	cytogenic fibrosing alveolitis
CFTR	cystic fibrosis transmembrane (conductance) regulator
CMV	cytomegalovirus
CNPA	chronic necrotizing pulmonary aspergillosis
COP	cryptogenic organizing pneumonitis
COPD	chronic obstructive pulmonary disease
CPAP	continuous positive airway pressure
CT	computerized tomography
CWP	coal workers pneumoconiosis
DOT	directly observed therapy
DPLD	diffuse parenchymal lung disease
DPT	diffuse pleural thickening
DTPA	diethylene triamine pentacetic acid
EAA	extrinsic allergic alveolitis
ECG	electrocardiogram
ECMO	extra corporeal membrane oxygenation
ESR	erythrocyte sedimentation rate
ETT	endotracheal tube
FA	fibrosing alveolitis
FASSc	fibrosing alveolitis in systemic sclerosis
FBC	full blood count
FEV_1	volume expired in first second of a forced expiration
FiO_2	inspired oxygen fraction
FOB	fibre-optic bronchoscopy
FRC	functional residual capacity
HFV	high frequency ventilation
HLA	histocompatibility leukocyte antigen
HPOA	hypertrophic pulmonary osteoarthropathy
HRCT	high resolution computerized tomography

I:E	inspiratory:expiratory
ILO	International Labour Organization
IPPV	intermittent positive pressure ventilation
IV	intravenous
IVOX	intravascular oxygenation
KCO	carbon monoxide transfer coefficient
KS	Kaposi's sarcoma
LAM	lymphangioleiomyomatosis
LCH	Langerhans cell histocytosis
LTOT	long-term oxygen therapy
LVRS	lung volume reduction surgery
MAI	*Mycobacterium avium intracellulaire*
MDR	multi-drug resistance
MK	*Mycobacterium kansasii*
MM	*Mycobacterium malmoense*
MR	magnetic resonance
MRI	magnetic resonance imaging
MTB	*Mycobacterium tuberculosis*
MX	*Mycobacterium xenopi*
NIPPV	nasal intermittent positive pressure ventilation
NPA	necrotizing pulmonary aspergillus
NSAIDs	non-steroidal anti-inflammatory drugs
OLB	open lung biopsy
OSA	obstructive sleep apnoea
PA	postero-anterior
PaO_2	arterial partial pressure of oxygen
$PaCO_2$	arterial partial pressure of carbon dioxide
PCNB	percutaneous needle biopsy
PCP	*Pneumocystis carinii* pneumonia
PEEP	positive end-expiratory pressure
PEFR	peak expiratory flow rate
PMF	progressive massive fibrosis
PO	oral
PPH	primary pulmonary hypertension
R/T	radiotherapy
RA	rheumatoid arthritis
RV	residual volume
SCLC	small-cell lung cancer
SIRS	systemic inflammatory response syndrome
SLE	systemic lupus erythematosus
SR	standardized residual
SVC	superior vena cava
SVCO	superior vena caval obstruction
TB	tuberculosis
TBB	transbronchial biopsy
TLC	total lung capacity
TLCO	carbon monoxide transfer factor

TPE	tropical pulmonary eosinophilia
V/Q	ventilation/perfusion
VATS	video-assisted thorascopic surgery
VC	vital capacity

PREFACE

This book is intended to be a concise guide to clinical respiratory medicine. The chapters are in a standard format, but vary in their approach from discussion of symptoms (e.g. Cough) to specific diseases (e.g. Sarcoidosis) to clinical scenarios (e.g. Immunodeficiency). Basic science topics – anatomy, physiology, pharmacology, immunology etc. – are only included in relation to specific clinical problems. In a book of this size it is not possible to cover every aspect of respiratory medicine, and for more detailed information on less common topics the reader is referred to more comprehensive texts.

We hope that this book will be useful to several different groups who wish to expand their knowledge of respiratory medicine. This will include trainees taking up a post on respiratory firm, and those responsible for admitting patients with acute respiratory problems in the course of a general medical take. Respiratory problems are a common reason for admission to the Intensive Care Unit, and those working in this area should also find this book of interest. Candidates for postgraduate examinations in Medicine (Parts 1 and 2 of the MRCP) will find all the necessary facts herein, and many of the topics relevant to exams in Anaesthesia.

We would like to thank John Duffy (Thoracic Surgical Techniques), Nick Sarkies (Clinical Examination), Lucy Speight (Clinical Examination) and Martin Wastie (Chest X-rays and Imaging Techniques) for helpful comments

ADULT RESPIRATORY DISTRESS SYNDROME

First described in 1967, the adult respiratory distress syndrome (ARDS) occurs secondary to lung injury from a wide range of insults. Variations in its definition have bedevilled the study of ARDS, and some authors term it 'Acute' rather than 'Adult' RDS.

ARDS is usually taken to include

- Clinical respiratory distress (more than 20 breaths per minute and laboured breathing).
- Diffuse infiltrates on the chest X-ray (CXR).
- PaO_2 less than 7.5 kPa when FiO_2 is greater than 50%.
- Normal pulmonary capillary wedge and plasma oncotic pressures.
- No clinical evidence of heart failure, fluid overload or chronic lung disease.
- Underlying associated condition.

Aetiology

The following factors are associated with development with ARDS

1. Direct lung injury.
- Aspiration of gastric contents.
- Infection (viral, bacterial, miliary TB).
- Inhalation of fumes/toxins (smoke, nitrogen oxides, oxygen).
- Trauma – lung contusion.
- Near-drowning.
- Radiation pneumonitis.

2. Indirect lung injury.
- Trauma.
- Sepsis.
- Multiple transfusions.
- Cardiopulmonary bypass.
- Acute pancreatitis.
- Disseminated intravascular coagulation.
- Drugs (heroin, salicylates).
- Fat embolism.
- Major burns.

Conditions that predispose to ARDS cause injury to the alveolar epithelium or vascular endothelium either directly (e.g. fume inhalation) or indirectly (e.g. sepsis). Trauma and sepsis account for approximately two-thirds of all cases.

Widely varying estimates of incidence have been reported, in part owing to difficulties in case definition. Annual rates between 2 and 75 per 10^5 population have been quoted. The lower figure is probably more realistic, coming from a population study over 3 years in Gran Canaria and broadly supported by studies elsewhere. It has been estimated that the average District General Hospital in the UK will see around 10–15 ARDS cases annually. The likelihood of developing ARDS is less than 25% with one predisposing factor, rising to over 80% with three factors.

The major sites of lung injury are the pulmonary endothelium and epithelium. Irrespective of the cause, there is an increase in neutrophils in bronchoalveolar lavage (BAL) fluid and a massive increase in protein permeability across the endothelium and epithelium. The pulmonary oedema protein concentration approaches that of plasma. These features occur in the first day of ARDS and persist for several days, following which there is a decline in both the proportion of neutrophils in BAL fluid and the protein concentration.

Both pro-inflammatory and anti-inflammatory cytokines are found in the lungs of ARDS patients starting in the 'at risk' period and persisting in those with prolonged disease. IL-1β and TNF-α contribute to initiation of inflammation, while levels of the neutrophil chemokine IL-8 in BAL fluid may predict patients going on to ARDS.

Histology shows pulmonary oedema and thrombi in engorged capillaries with development of hyaline membrane formation. In survivors interstitial fibrosis may develop. Patients with ARDS suffer severe gas exchange abnormalities with increased ventilation/perfusion mismatch and increased intrapulmonary shunting. Compliance falls (stiff lungs) with a reduction in functional residual capacity (FRC) of up to 50%. The development of pulmonary hypertension further reduces cardiac output. Peripheral oxygen uptake is often low in critically ill patients, even if PaO_2 is restored to normal.

Clinical features

The first signs of ARDS, breathlessness and tachypnoea, begin 12–48 h after the onset of the insult. The CXR shows bilateral diffuse infiltrates. Unlike cardiogenic pulmonary oedema, there is no cardiac enlargement or septal (Kerley) lines and effusions are rare. The patient is hypoxaemic (see definition) and usually hypocapnic with a pulmonary capillary wedge pressure less than 18 mm Hg.

Management

1. *Underlying cause.* Treatment of the predisposing factor(s) is obviously essential.

2. *Ventilation and oxygenation.* Many patients may be managed with continuous positive airway pressure (CPAP) via a face mask, with the advantages of retained consciousness and avoidance of the adverse effects of ventilation on cardiac output. If PaO_2 remains lower than 8 kPa, full ventilatory support is likely to be necessary. With mechanical ventilation it is important to use the lowest FiO_2 and airway pressure to achieve a balance between adequate oxygenation (at least 85% oxygen saturation, preferably 90%) and adverse effects from ventilation.

The use of PEEP (positive end-expiratory pressure) at 5–15 cm H_2O improves oxygenation, probably by increasing

FRC and alveolar recruitment of collapsed lung units. The major adverse effects of PEEP are barotrauma (e.g. pneumothorax, interstitial emphysema) and reduced cardiac output owing to reduced venous return and increased right ventricular afterload.

Lengthening inspiratory time (increased I:E ratio) is used with PEEP to set the mean airway pressure while limiting peak airway pressure. In about half of all patients, turning to the prone position improves oxygenation sufficiently to allow reduced PEEP or FiO_2, but there have been no controlled trials of this manoeuvre. High frequency ventilation (HFV) appears to improve oxygenation via increasing mean airway pressure, but there has been no survival benefit in controlled studies.

In contrast with methods of ventilation that recruit alveolar units but which may damage the lung, others have proposed resting the lung ('recruitment vs. rest'). Tolerating a higher $PaCO_2$ (permissive hypercapnia) has its proponents. Extra corporeal membrane oxygenation (ECMO) showed no benefit in a controlled study in 1994. Devices have been developed to provide intravascular oxygenation (IVOX) but at best provide less than 50% basal oxygen requirements – again trials have not shown improved outcome.

3. Fluid balance, circulation and nutrition. The dramatic increase in lung permeability provides a rationale for keeping the circulating volume low. Diuretics, fluid restriction and, on occasions, dialysis or ultrafiltration may be used to keep the wedge pressure down to around 8–10 mm Hg. Cardiac output may then need inotropic support rather than volume replacement. However, there are no definite data on outcome with the use of 'drying out' and inotropic support.

Peripheral oxygen delivery is maximal with an Hb of approximately 12 g/dl. Metabolic abnormalities should be corrected. An inappropriately low systemic vascular resistance can lead to poor perfusion of vital organs, and a peripheral vasoconstrictor such as noradrenaline should be considered. Care must be taken with parenteral nutrition because of the associated fluid load.

4. Systemic treatments. The systemic inflammatory response syndrome (SIRS) frequently occurs in ARDS. Three randomized studies of steroids in ARDS have, however, been negative. Steroids currently have no role in routine management. A controlled study of the anti-oxidant N-acetylcysteine showed no benefit. Ketoconazole is a potent inhibitor of thromboxane A_2, and a small study showed improved mortality. Trials are being undertaken of inhibitors of the adhesion molecules associated with neutrophil ingress into tissues.

5. *Local treatments.* Inhaled nitric oxide dilates pulmonary vessels in ventilated areas with resulting reduction in pulmonary artery pressure and intrapulmonary shunting. Results of trials on outcome are awaited.

There has been immense interest in surfactant, which is a mixture of phospholipids, neutral lipids and unique surfactant proteins. Surfactant lines the gas–liquid interface and reduces surface tension and the work of breathing with anti-oxidant and anti-inflammatory activity. Artificial surfactant is routinely used in neo-natal RDS, supported by clinical trials. In ARDS oedema fluid proteins inhibit the surface properties of surfactant, and proteases and oxygen radicals affect surfactant protein, leading to decreased quantity and function of the material. The first trial of surfactant in ARDS showed no benefit in 30-day survival in sepsis-induced ARDS. Unfortunately, the artificial surfactant used did not contain surfactant proteins and other studies are being performed.

Outcome

Mortality remains at around 50%. Most patients with ARDS die, though not directly from it, the usual cause of death being multi-organ failure. There is no reliable indicator of outcome amongst the various indicators of severity of ARDS. Serum ferritin may predict which patients will develop ARDS, but larger studies are needed.

In survivors, approximately 50% have breathlessness and cough at 1 year though only 10–15% have disability. Over 50% of survivors have reduced gas transfer at 1 year whilst spirometry tends to return to normal. Most patients with persisting abnormalities have restrictive lung function, but a small group have airflow obstruction. There is no agreement on whether a high FiO_2 affects lung function in survivors.

Further reading

Badouin SV. Surfactant medication for acute respiratory distress syndrome. *Thorax* 1997; **52** (supp 13): S9–S15.

Beale R. Grover ER, Smithies M, et al. Acute respiratory distress syndrome ('ARDS'): no more than a severe acute lung injury. *British Medical Journal* 1993; **307:** 1335–1339.

Related topic of interest

ASBESTOS

Asbestos is a general term for fibrous silicates. Amphiboles are straight stiff fibres, for example crocidolite (blue asbestos) and amosite (brown asbestos), while serpentine fibres are flexible and curly, for example chrysotile (white asbestos). Asbestos is used for its fire and electrical resistance and mechanical strength.

Occupations with substantial asbestos exposure include

- Laggers.
- Boiler men.
- Trades involved with insulation, fire proofing and cladding of buildings.
- Ship building trades.
- Asbestos textile industry.
- Friction material workers, for example brake linings.
- Joiners, electricians, plumbers, power station workers, demolition workers.

Environmental exposures may affect those living close to asbestos factories or in regions of Turkey where there is a high incidence of asbestos-related disease owing to naturally occurring zeolite. The risks of incidental exposure to asbestos in buildings create public concern but are minute and negligible in comparison with many other risks, for example drowning, accidents, or smoking. Some dangers of asbestos were well known by the 1940s. However, in the UK it was not until the early 1970s, following the 1969 Asbestos Industry Regulations, that adequate work-force protection became usual.

Pleural plaques

Plaques are discrete, irregular, fibrotic, often calcified, lesions on the parietal pleura, diaphragm and pericardium. The pathogenesis is not understood. Asbestos fibres are rarely found in the pleural space. Up to 50% of people exposed to asbestos (mainly to amphiboles) will have calcified pleural plaques after 30 years. There is a broad relationship with cumulative doses. Plaques are, however, occasionally found after minimal exposure.

Plaques are almost always symptomless, usually found incidentally on a CXR. There is no effect on lung function. Very rarely with extensive plaques there may be shortness of breath or pain. On CXR, plaques appear as protuberances on the lateral chest wall, or linear calcification on the diaphragm. Calcified plaques seen *en face* show an irregular 'holly leaf' or 'candle grease' pattern. A CT scan is helpful when there is doubt but is not needed routinely.

Plaques may increase in size for some years after exposure ceases, but have no effect on survival. There is no evidence that plaques progress to other pleural disease including mesothelioma. The extent of asbestos exposure determines the risk of other asbestos-related disease, irrespective of the extent of plaques.

Pleural effusion

Possibly up to 20% of asbestos-exposed workers develop an effusion at some time but, as these are usually asymptomatic, the true frequency is difficult to estimate. Effusions usually occur less than 20 years after initial exposure and are normally small, though there may be pleuritic pain. About 50% are blood stained. Spontaneous resolution is normal, though CXR usually shows a blunted costophrenic angle. Some workers develop diffuse pleural thickening (DPT; see below).

Diffuse pleural thickening

The prevalence of DPT in exposed workers is approximately 5%. DPT is more closely related to cumulative doses than is pleural plaques. DPT may be asymptomatic or cause breathlessness owing to a restrictive effect. It may follow episodes of pleurisy, but pain is uncommon with established DPT. CXR usually shows bilateral symmetrical mid-zone thickening with obliterated costophrenic angles. Frequently, fibrous strands extend from the pleura (crow's feet appearance). Lung function shows a restrictive defect with reduced total lung capacity (TLC) and carbon monoxide transfer factor (TLCO) but a raised carbon monoxide transfer coefficient (KCO) (owing to lung squashing effect).

The diagnosis is usually clinical and requires an appropriate history of asbestos exposure, and exclusion of other causes of pleural thickening (e.g. TB, connective tissue disorder, drugs, trauma). Biopsy may be necessary to exclude mesothelioma particularly if the thickening is unilateral. If disabling symptoms are present, decortication should be considered. DPT may progress after exposure stops; it does not progress to mesothelioma but the exposure necessary to cause DPT is itself associated with increased risks of mesothelioma, lung cancer and asbestosis.

Mesothelioma

Mesothelioma is a malignant neoplasm of the pleura (or peritoneum, less commonly). The causal link with asbestos was established in 1960. About 85% of cases have a history of asbestos exposure. Mesothelioma is much more likely after amphibole exposure than chrysotile. Asbestos may be a direct carcinogen, but other co-factors could be involved. There is current interest in the possible role of Simian virus 40 which contaminated polio vaccine in the 1950s–1960s. The risk of mesothelioma increases with dose and with time from exposure. It is not related to cigarette smoking. The mean latent period between first exposure to asbestos and mesothelioma is around 35–40 years; it rarely occurs under 20 years. The incidence of mesothelioma is rising and will peak between 2010 and 2020 when it may account for up to 1% of male deaths in the UK.

1. Clinical features. Breathlessness and chest pain are usual. Breathlessness is often initially due to pleural effusion (>80%), and later to tumour encasing the lung. Chest pain is often severe. Ascites or intestinal obstruction occur with peritoneal involvement. Clinical signs are those of pleural effusion or thickening. Tumour masses often track through biopsy or drain sites. Clubbing is unusual (<10%). Pericardial constriction may occur.

2. *Investigations.* CXR shows one or more of
- Pleural effusion, usually unilateral.
- Lobulated pleural opacities.
- Spread of tumour into fissures.
- Markers of asbestos exposure, e.g. calcified pleural plaques, are present in a majority.

The effusion is blood stained in one-third of cases. It is difficult to distinguish malignant from reactive mesothelial cells in pleural fluid cytology. Closed pleural biopsy reveals the diagnosis in only approximately 50% owing to small samples, but is usually done to exclude other conditions. Thoracoscopy provides larger samples and a diagnosis in approximately 90%.

Mesothelioma spreads over the pleural surface to encase the lung, invading the fissures and pericardium. It may involve the peritoneum and liver. Histology varies from the sarcomatous type to epithelial type. The latter is often difficult to distinguish from secondary adenocarcinoma. Immunohistochemical stains are increasingly helpful. Distant metastases occur in over one-third of cases, but are not often clinically evident.

3. *Treatment.* Surgery is very occasionally performed for early disease but its efficacy is not known and trials are awaited. Chemical pleurodesis or recurrent aspiration is useful for control of effusion, and palliative radiotherapy for painful chest-wall tumour masses. Pain relief is frequently difficult and may require specialist involvement.

4. *Outcome.* Median survival is 12–18 months from presentation. There is no evidence that current therapy affects survival. There are ongoing trials of chemotherapy and proposed trials of radical surgery.

Asbestosis

Asbestosis is lung fibrosis resulting from asbestos exposure. The period between the start of exposure and symptoms is usually 20 years or more. Heavy exposure is usually required before asbestosis develops. Individual susceptibility is likely to be important in determining whether the accumulation of asbestos fibres in alveolar macrophages triggers subsequent inflammation and fibrosis.

1. *Clinical features.* The symptoms are those of pulmonary fibrosis. A gradual onset of breathlessness on exertion is usual.

A cough productive of mucoid sputum is common. Haemoptysis or pain suggest lung cancer or mesothelioma, respectively.

Finger clubbing is uncommon in early disease and even in late disease occurs in less than 50%. Fine late-inspiratory bilateral basal crackles are characteristic of pulmonary fibrosis and may precede CXR abnormalities. In later disease crackles may be heard throughout inspiration and subsequently in expiration.

2. *Investigations and diagnosis.* CXR shows predominantly basal and symmetrical linear and irregular opacities. However, up to 20% of patients with histologically proved asbestosis have a normal CXR. About 75% of patients with asbestosis have coexistent pleural change (plaques or DPT). CT scanning reveals sub-pleural lines, parenchymal bands, and later findings of fibrosis (septal thickening and honeycombing). All these findings are non-specific, though parenchymal bands are probably commoner in asbestosis than cryptogenic fibrosing alveolitis (CFA). High resolution computerized tomography (HRCT) scanning is more sensitive than CXR and is useful in the presence of symptoms and/or lung function impairment with a normal or equivocal CXR, or when extensive pleural abnormality makes it difficult to differentiate pleural and parenchymal disease.

Lung function tests are those of pulmonary fibrosis, that is a restrictive defect with preserved FEV/VC ratio, reduced lung volumes, and reduced gas transfer and KCO. If there is also significant pleural disease the KCO may be normal or increased.

Asbestos bodies are asbestos fibres coated with ferritin, and are found in sputum, BAL fluid or histological specimens. Such bodies are markers of previous asbestos exposure, but their presence or absence neither proves nor refutes disease resulting from asbestos. Although asbestosis is usually a clinical diagnosis, a biopsy may be required (either thoracoscopically or at post-mortem) where there is doubt. A count of asbestos fibres (using electron microscopy) quantifies the asbestos burden and can support a diagnosis of asbestosis.

A diagnosis of asbestosis is made by

- An appropriate history of exposure, i.e. at least moderate asbestos exposure for several years.
- Appropriate clinical features including breathlessness and late inspiratory basal crackles.
- Restrictive lung function and compatible CXR.
- Exclusion of other diffuse parenchymal lung diseases particularly CFA.

3. *Treatment and outcome.* In modern times the disease usually progresses slowly or is stable. The risk of progression

is related to cumulative dose, amphibole exposure, early onset of disease, clubbing, and possibly to smoking. In progressive disease treatment should probably be as for CFA, but there have been no treatment trials. Of patients certified as having asbestosis, one study indicated that 39% died of lung cancer, 20% of asbestosis and 9% of mesothelioma.

Lung cancer

It has been known since the mid-1950s that the risk of lung cancer is increased by asbestos exposure, especially for amphiboles. There is a long-running debate as to whether a threshold of asbestos exposure must be exceeded before the risk of lung cancer increases. The current majority expert view is that there is indeed a threshold, and that lung cancer can only be ascribed to asbestos exposure when asbestosis is also present. Smoking and asbestos together exert a synergistic effect on the increased risk of lung cancer. The investigation, pathology, and treatment of lung cancer is similar in patients with and without asbestosis.

Rounded atelectasis

Pseudotumour, rounded atelectasis, Blesovsky's syndrome, and folded lung are synonyms for a condition in which focal lung collapse with infolding is secondary to an area of underlying pleural fibrosis. A rounded opacity is produced suggesting a tumour, but biopsy shows fibrosis. The CT scan shows curving vessels and bronchi going into the edge of the lesion. The syndrome is not specific to asbestos-related pleural disease but may also occur after other causes of pleural fibrosis, including empyema and trauma.

Compensation

In many countries, state-funded compensation is available. In the UK compensation is available for mesothelioma, asbestosis, bilateral DPT and lung cancer, provided the latter occurs in the presence of asbestosis or DPT. The claimant does not have to prove negligence, merely a history of exposure and the presence of disease. A civil action in respect of these conditions and for pleural plaques may be successful where it can be proved that an employer failed to protect workers despite knowledge of asbestos-related effects. In the UK all cases in which a patient's death is thought to relate to asbestos exposure should be reported to the Coroner.

Further reading

Parkes WR. *Occupational lung disorders*. Oxford: Butterworth, 1994.

Related topics of interest

ASPERGILLUS

Micheli, a botanist and priest, named this fungus aspergillus in 1729 because its spore-bearing heads were similar in appearance to the aspergillum used to scatter holy water. *Aspergillus fumigatus* is the most important human pathogen, although there are more than 130 other species, some of which (e.g. *Aspergillus flavus, niger, terreus*) occasionally cause disease. Aspergillus spores can be recovered from both indoor and many outdoor environments, with an increased concentration in winter. Spores are around 3 μm in diameter and therefore easily lodge in the terminal bronchioles in the lung.

Aspergillus almost always causes disease in the presence of underlying lung disease (e.g. asthma, fibrosis, cavities or immunosuppression). The spectrum of disease is wide but can be subdivided as follows:

- *Colonization*: aspergilloma.
- *Allergic*: positive skin tests, asthma, allergic bronchopulmonary aspergillosis (ABPA), extrinsic allergic alveolitis, bronchocentric granulomatosis.
- *Invasive*: invasive aspergillosis, chronic necrotizing pulmonary aspergillosis (CNPA).

Aspergilloma

Aspergillus spores can be found in sputum without definite evidence of tissue damage (saprophytic disease). This usually occurs in chronic lung disease such as bronchiectasis or cystic fibrosis (CF). It can be difficult to distinguish colonization from disease. An aspergilloma is a fungal ball developing in a pre-existing cavity. About 25% patients with aspergilloma have a history of tuberculosis, the most common predisposing cause. Aspergillomas can also develop in lungs affected by sarcoidosis, lung cysts, ankylosing spondylitis, etc. Aspergillomas are usually single, but are multiple in approximately 20%. In a 1970 study 17% of patients with old tuberculous cavities had evidence of aspergilloma after a minimum 4 year follow-up period.

1. Clinical features. An aspergilloma may be an asymptomatic CXR finding. Patients may present with haemoptysis (about 75%) owing to erosion of a bronchial artery, cough and sputum or systemic symptoms, for example fever, malaise, weight loss. Finger clubbing is rare.

2. Investigations. The classic CXR shows a dense opacity surrounded by a halo or crescent of air. The fungal ball varies with position. Pleural thickening over the cavity commonly precedes the development of the fungal ball. An aspergilloma can be demonstrated by CT scan if the CXR is not definitive. The differential includes cavitating neoplasm or pulmonary embolus, hydatid, pulmonary abscess. Serum precipitins are found in nearly 100%, while skin-prick tests are only positive in 30%.

3. Management. For patients with debilitating symptoms, repeated hospital admission, or haemoptysis, the treatment of choice in a reasonably fit patient is surgery, with either lobar resection or cavernostomy. Some authors also suggest early surgery, before the progression of lung disease and comorbidities, but there is no direct evidence for this approach. Selection of patients is vital. In earlier surgical series, mortality was up to 25% but in modern series, mortality has ranged from 2 to 10% and morbidity at 20% (bleeding or fistulae).

With associated chronic lung disease, many patients are not fit for surgery. Unfortunately, medical management has limited success. Several uncontrolled series suggest that antifungal treatment (e.g. amphotericin or potassium iodide) via a catheter placed into the cavity both improves symptoms and reduces haemoptysis, though cannot cure. Oral itraconazole has a variable effect and there are no controlled trials. Corticosteroids help malaise but must be used cautiously in view of the possibility of inducing invasive disease.

4. Outcome. Ten percent of aspergillomas resolve spontaneously. Between 2 and 20% of patients with aspergilloma are reported to die from haemopytsis.

Allergic broncho-pulmonary aspergillosis

ABPA, first described in 1952, is the commonest cause of pulmonary eosinophilia in the UK. Almost all ABPA is associated with asthma, but only 1% of asthmatics get ABPA. It also occurs in 10% of patients with CF. There is no apparent increase in exposure to aspergillus spores in those with ABPA compared with asthmatics without ABPA. ABPA is a hypersensitive reaction to spores of aspergillus. Both IgE and IgG antibodies play a major role in pathogenesis. The process mainly involves the bronchial wall and peripheral lung, but without dissemination.

1. Diagnostic criteria. Variable diagnostic criteria have been used but generally include:
- History of asthma.
- Eosinophilia ($>0.5 \times 10^9$ per litre).
- Pulmonary infiltrates on CXR.
- Positive skin test to *Aspergillus fumigatus*.
- Raised total IgE, and precipitins to *Aspergillus fumigatus*.

Fungal hyphae in sputum are supportive of the diagnosis.

2. Pathology and pathogenesis. The airways contain mucous plugs containing aspergillus hyphae with distal collapse. There is little or no evidence of invasion of the bronchial wall or parenchyma. In acute ABPA with pulmonary infiltrates there is pulmonary eosinophilia. A mononuclear cell infiltrate and granulomata, as well as eosinophilic infiltrate and giant cells, suggest a cell-mediated reaction.

A positive skin test to *Aspergillus fumigatus* is common in asthmatics and in such patients inhalation of aspergillus spores may precipitate asthma exacerbation. Why a minority of aspergillus-sensitive asthmatics develop ABPA is not known. Host susceptibility may be important, though no genetic predisposition has yet been identified.

3. Clinical features. ABPA occurs in asthmatics at any age and presents usually with worsening asthma, increased purulent sputum, fever, and sometimes coughing bronchial plugs of fungal mycelia.

4. Investigations. The CXR in acute ABPA shows diffuse perihilar infiltrates which are often transient or fleeting, and collapse. Eosinophilia is invariable and may be very high with pulmonary infiltrates (typically at 1.0–3.0 per 10^9). Finding of aspergillus in sputum is only supportive, though hyphae suggest the growth of aspergillus in bronchi. A positive skin test to aspergillus is common in asthmatics generally and in CF, but is a prerequisite for the diagnosis of ABPA. Total IgE is higher than in asthma, owing to an increase in both non-specific and specific IgE. Aspergillus precipitins (IgG) are found in two-thirds of patients with ABPA in undiluted serum but up to 90% in concentrated serum. Their presence does not reflect disease activity and neither does the level of specific IgG. Precipitins are also found in up to 18% of asthmatics and 30% of CF sufferers without ABPA.

Bronchiectasis is a result of chronic disease. Typically in ABPA this involves proximal and upper lobe bronchi – other types of bronchiectasis are more often distal. In chronic ABPA the CXR shows upper zone tramlining, with gloved finger projections owing to mucus impaction in dilated bronchi. HRCT shows proximal bronchiectasis and chronic upper zone fibrosis. In a recent study, bronchiectasis was found with HRCT in 85% of 134 lobes in 23 patients at diagnosis.

5. Management. Steroids are first line therapy and inhibit aspergillus growth, decreasing sputum volume and reversing pulmonary infiltration and systemic symptoms. They are not fungicidal. The recommended regime is 40 mg daily tapering according to a response over 3 months. Some authors suggest that monitoring IgE and CXR for infiltrates with appropriate prednisolone therapy *may* prevent progression to bronchiectasis. For patients with frequent exacerbations, a daily maintainance dose of 10 mg is often necessary. Low-dose inhaled steroids are ineffective. Some reports suggest disease control with higher dose inhaled steroids in some patients. Uncontrolled trials suggest that itraconazole may have a steroid-sparing role in steroid-dependent patients. If lobar segmental collapse does not respond to high-dose prednisolone, broncho-dilators and physiotherapy, bronchoscopy should be performed to remove mucus plugs.

6. Outcome. ABPA often follows a chronic relapsing course. With current therapy, progression to bronchiectasis seems likely in the majority of patients despite the use of steroids.

Invasive aspergillosis

Invasive aspergillosis almost always affects immuno-compromised patients. There is an increasing incidence because of the larger numbers of patients with such disease. Any immuno-suppressed patient is at risk but high risk groups are:

- Acute leukaemia, lymphoma.
- Neutropenia.
- Solid organ transplant.
- Bone marrow transplant.
- Chronic granulomatous disease.

The disease is rare in AIDS, unless there are other factors such as steroids, neutropenia, etc.

1. Pathology. Aspergillus hyphae invade bronchial walls and surrounding lung to cause a necrotizing pneumonia. Invasion of blood vessels causes thrombosis and infarction. Invasive aspergillosis usually affects the lung parenchyma, but airway disease can predominate with tracheo-bronchial ulcers or pseudomembraneous tracheo-bronchitis.

2. Clinical features. Pulmonary disease is the commonest presentation of invasive aspergillosis. Thus, fever and non-specific pulmonary infiltrates (owing to necrotizing pneumonia) are the commonest presentation. Pleuritic chest pain, haemoptysis and pleural rub (owing to pulmonary infarction) may occur. Pulmonary haemorrhage is rare. The lung disease may lead to disseminated aspergillosis (cerebral, osteomyelitis, endocarditis, sinusitis), but occasionally this also occurs without pulmonary involvement.

3. Investigations. The CXR is often non-specific, showing infiltrates or one or more rounded solid or cavitating shadows. The CT is of great help – the finding of an irregular halo around a nodular shadow is sufficiently predictive of invasive aspergillosis to initiate treatment. The halo sign precedes cavitation or the crescent sign. The latter is seen in late disease usually with an increase in white cell count.

Culture of aspergillus in sputum or BAL fluid is insensitive, but in a neutropenic patient a positive aspergillus culture is highly predictive (about 90%) for invasive disease. The predictive value of an aspergillus culture is much lower in other clinical situations. Diagnostic yield at fibre-optic bronchoscopy (FOB) is at least 50%, but many patients are too ill for such invasive procedures. Antibodies to aspergillus have lower sensitivity and specificity and are unhelpful clinically.

4. *Management.* Treatment needs to begin early. Amphotericin (1 mg/kg/day) in neutropenic and BMT patients should be given with flucytosine (200 mg/kg/day). A lower dose of amphotericin (0.7 mg) with or without flucytosine is recommended for other patients. Amphotericin has synergistic nephrotoxicity with cyclosporin. However, as lower doses of amphotericin may be ineffective, liposomal amphotericin is indicated in this situation. Studies suggest that early treatment may bring mortality down to 50%. In less immunocompromized patients itraconazole (200 mg/day) has good activity.

Chronic necrotizing pulmonary aspergillosis

This is a more indolent form of invasive disease. Fever and a productive cough are common and may occur for weeks, months or years. CNPA occurs in patients with pre-existing pulmonary disease (e.g. ankylosing spondylitis or diabetes). CXR shows infiltrative cavitating disease, sometimes with a fungal ball. Pathology is that of aspergillus hyphae invading lung parenchyma but without disseminated aspergillosis.

Itraconazole has documented efficacy and low toxicity, though there are no controlled trials. It is recommended that itraconazole (200 mg/day) is given for a month and continued if there is improvement. If there is no improvement, surgery should be considered but if the patient is not fit then amphotericin should be tried at 0.7 mg/kg/day.

Bronchocentric granulomatosis

This is a necrotizing granulomatous process of peripheral airways. Most asthmatics are hypersensitive to *Aspergillus fumigatus*, but in non-asthmatics a variety of other antigens are found or the aetiology is unknown. It usually presents either as an asymptomatic nodule(s) or with low-grade fever, weight loss and cough. Diagnosis is often made after surgery for suspected tumour. CXR may show nodules, infiltrates or bronchiectasis.

Further reading

Elliott MW, Newman Taylor AJ. Allergic broncho-pulmonary aspergillosis. *Clin. Exp. Allergy.* 1997; **27**(suppl 1):55–59.

Gordon IJ, Evans CC. Aspergillus lung disease. *Journal of the Royal College of Physicians* 1986; **20**: 206–211.

Wilson M, Denning DW. The commonest life-threatening mould infections: invasive aspergillosis. *Hospital Update* **1993**: 225–233.

Related topics of interest

ASTHMA

Asthma remains the most important cause of morbidity due to respiratory disease in children and young adults. The prevalence is about 10–14% in the UK and wheezing illness has increased in prevalence over the last 20 years in most westernized populations. There is no universally agreed definition of the disease, but the American Thoracic Society definition requires:

(a) Symptoms (cough, wheeze or breathlessness).
(b) Either day to day variability in mean peak flow rates >15% or reversibility to inhaled β_2 agonists >20%.
(c) Airway hyper-responsiveness (qv).

Pathologically, asthma is best described as a *chronic eosinophilic bronchitis.*

Aetiology

Asthma occurs in a given individual owing to a combination of *genetic predisposition* and exposure to the appropriate *environmental stimulus.*

1. Genetic predisposition. The heritable component of the disease is likely to be due to the influence of a number of different genes; linkage of asthma or surrogates for asthma (total IgE, bronchial hyper-responsiveness, atopy) has been demonstrated on chromosome 5 (to the Th_2 cytokine cluster), chromosome 11 (to the FcεR1 high affinity IgE receptor locus) and chromosome 12.

2. Environmental stimuli. Include maternal smoking, lack of exposure to childhood infection, exposure to high concentrations of allergens (house dust mite in the UK, cockroach in the USA), eating a refined diet high in salt and low in magnesium, and exposure to sensitizers and irritants at work (see below).

3. Disease prevalence has increased over the last 20 years in the west; currently 1 in 7 school children will be diagnosed as asthmatic and as many as 1 in 3 will wheeze at some stage. The increase cannot be accounted for by genetic factors and must be due to altered environmental exposure to precipitants.

4. Air pollution. Components of air pollution (particulates (PM_{10}), ozone and nitrogen oxides) can cause exacerbation of asthma but there is no good evidence that air pollution causes asthma *per se.*

Pathology

1. Bronchial biopsies from patients with asthma reveal inflammatory changes in both the large and small airways. Typically there is a Th_2 mediated inflammatory response with increased numbers of eosinophils, mast cells and small increases in T-cell and macrophage numbers. Increased numbers of cells stain for Th_2 cytokines (eg interleukin 4,5). There is thickening of the basement membrane with epithelial desquamation.

2. *Airway remodelling* occurs in chronic disease with hypertrophy and hyperplasia of smooth muscle and subepithelial fibrosis.

Clinical features

1. *Symptoms and signs.* Typical symptoms are cough, wheeze and occasionally exercise-related breathlessness. There is marked variability in the ability of patients to judge the severity of their bronchospasm. Expiratory wheeze may or may not be present on examination when the patient is well.

Peak flow monitoring reveals peak flow variability, frequently with morning dips, and reversibility to inhaled bronchodilators. Spot peak flow measurements are unreliable in diagnosis. Markers for poor asthma control include increasing symptoms, nocturnal awakening with cough or wheeze, increasing use of bronchodilator medication and either increased peak flow variability or a fall in mean peak flow values.

Sub-phenotypes of asthma

A number of different groups of asthmatics have been identified and, although these overlap, the characteristics of these groups are given below.

1. *Extrinsic asthma.* Young patients who are atopic (i.e. who have positive skin-prick tests to common allergens) and have elevated IgE levels and frequently associated symptoms from eczema or allergic rhinitis. Symptoms often remit after the age of 15 but may recur later in life.

2. *Intrinsic asthma.* Older patients (>30 years), often with no clear history of atopy. Skin tests are usually negative and IgE levels within the normal range. Spontaneous remission is rare.

3. *Occupational asthma.* A large range of sensitizers and irritants at work can precipitate asthma in susceptible individuals (*Table 1*). Occupational asthma should be suspected in exposed individuals with work-related symptoms (although there may be delay of several hours between exposure and symptom onset). Symptoms typically improve at weekends and on holiday. Investigation of choice is 2 hourly peak-flow monitoring with diary record cards. If exposure continues, the disease may become chronic (even if later exposure ceases), but early (< 2 years) removal from exposure may lead to complete remission.

4. *Aspirin-induced asthma.* Patients in whom exposure to aspirin and other non-steroidal anti-inflammatory agents can precipitate severe life-threatening bronchospasm. Prevalence

Table 1. Some causes of occupational asthma

Precipitent	Occupation
Animal proteins (e.g. excreta)	Laboratory workers
Shellfish proteins	Seafood workers
Grain/flour	Bakers
Fungi	Brewers
Isocyonates	Paint sprayers
Reactive dyes	Manufacturing
Acid anhydrides	Manufacturing
Drugs & enzymes	Pharmaceutical workers
Plicatic acid (Western Red Cedar)	Forestry workers
Pinewood resin (colophony)	Joiners

has been estimated to be as high as 5% but in non-specialist centres is probably less than 1%. Desensitization to aspirin produces short-term improvement but should only be performed by experienced practitioners.

5. Nocturnal asthma. Some patients demonstrate marked falls of peak flow rates at night accompanied with severe symptoms.

Treatment

National guidelines exist both in the UK and the USA for the treatment of patients with asthma and are summarized in *Table 2*. All patients should have inhaler technique assessed and the best inhaler device defined. Home peak-flow monitoring and self-management plans may improve asthma control.

Table 2. National guidelines for the treatment of patients with asthma

Disease severity	Step	Treatment
Mild	1	Short acting β2 agonist as required
	2	Regular inhaled steroid (<400 mcg/day beclomethasone or equivalent) plus Step 1
Moderate	3	Either high dose inhaled steroid plus Step 1, or Step 2 plus regular long acting β2 agonist
	4	High dose inhaled steroid plus Step 3, plus trial of other agents (theophylline, anticholinergic, cromolyn, high dose bronchodilator)
Severe	5	As step 4 plus regular oral steroid

1. Steroid-reducing measures. Many agents have been studied in an attempt to reduce requirements for oral steroids in patients with severe chronic asthma. Examples include theophyllines, cromoglycate, nedocromil, immunosuppressant agents (e.g. cyclosporin and methotrexate), nebulized steroids and anticholinergics. In general, most of these agents have a small effect but many patients in the group with severe disease still require regular treatment with oral steroids. Secondary prevention for osteoporosis should be considered for patients (especially post-menopausal women) on long-term oral steroids (HRT, bisphosphonates).

2. Leukotriene receptor antagonists. Two LTD4 antagonists (montelukast, zafirlukast) have been shown to be effective oral agents: their exact place in treatment protocols remains to be defined.

Acute exacerbations

Acute exacerbations can be triggered by coexistent viral respiratory tract infection, exposure to respiratory irritants (smoke, dust, allergens, air pollution), exercise, allergy and poor compliance with prophylactic treatment. Treatment of an acute attack is covered by national guidelines in the UK; and consists of oxygen, nebulized β_2 agonist and either intravenous or oral steroid (depending on severity). Intravenous aminophylline or β_{2x}-agonists and ventilatory support may be needed in severe cases.

Prognosis

Most patients with asthma have mild disease and never require hospital admission. About 2000 people each year die of asthma in the UK.

Bronchial hyper-reactivity

Bronchial hyper-reactivity is an inappropriate bronchoconstrictor response to an inhaled challenge. Measurement of airway reactivity is usually performed by administering incremental doses of a stimulus (usually histamine or methacholine, occasionally adenosine, cold air or allergen) and measuring change in FEV_1 from baseline. Subjects are deemed to be hyper-responsive if they drop their FEV_1 greater than 20% base line after inhalation of a set amount of irritant. The dose of irritant required to drop the FEV_1 by 20% is known as the PD20 (provocative dose causing a 20% fall in FEV_1).

1. Airway hyper-responsiveness (bronchial hyper-reactivity) occurs in the majority of patients with asthma (but not all) and may be present also in otherwise asymptomatic individuals and in association with other airway disease (e.g. CF).

Further reading

The British Guidelines on Asthma Management. *Thorax,* 1997; **52** supplement 1, pp. 1–21.
Hall IP. The future of asthma. *British Medical Journal,* 1997; **314:** 45–49.

Related topics of interest

Aspergillus (p. 11)
Chronic obstructive pulmonary disease (p. 37)
Pneumoconiosis (p. 120)
Pulmonary eosinophilia (p. 137)

BIOPSY TECHNIQUES

Obtaining material for cytology or histology is central to the diagnosis of many respiratory diseases, particularly malignancy. Bronchoscopic and thoracoscopic techniques are dealt with under the topics 'Fibre-optic bronchoscopy' and 'Thoracic surgical procedures'. This topic covers percutaneous biopsy of the lung, lymph nodes, or pleura.

Lymph node aspiration/biopsy

Formal excision biopsy of a cervical or axillary lymph node usually requires a general anaesthetic, and will almost certainly give a precise histological diagnosis in almost any disease. Samples of a resected node should always be sent in normal saline for mycobacterial culture.

A simpler technique is aspiration under local anaesthesia. This will often give a diagnosis in metastatic malignancy more quickly and with less discomfort for the patient than excision biopsy. The skin is infiltrated with 2% lignocaine using a syringe and orange (25G) needle. A white (19G) needle is attached to a 20 ml syringe and the tip passed through the skin. Suction is then applied by pulling out the plunger of the syringe. The needle is passed though the node several times, maintaining the suction throughout. The suction is then released, prior to withdrawal of the needle through the skin. The needle is detached from the syringe, and the material within the hollow bore of the needle is expelled onto a microscope slide by pushing air though the needle using the syringe. A second slide is then drawn along the first to make a smear, which can be fixed or air-dried depending upon the preference of the cytologist.

Percutaneous lung biopsy

In a patient with a CXR shadow thought to be a lung cancer, there is often debate about whether a percutaneous needle biopsy (PCNB) or a bronchoscopy is more likely to give the diagnosis. In general, a peripheral lesion is suitable for percutaneous biopsy, but one that is adjacent to the hilum is better approached with a bronchoscope. Bronchoscopy may be chosen as the initial investigation of a peripheral lesion if it is not well circumscribed or if there is a history of haemoptysis. In some centres, bronchoscopic biopsy forceps are passed into a peripheral lesion under radiographic screening with good diagnostic yields.

Radiographic screening is the most common way of localizing the lesion for percutaneous biopsy, but for some lesions CT may be necessary. After anaesthetizing the chest wall and pleura, a fine needle is introduced into the lesion. Depending upon the type of needle used, material for cytology or histology may be obtained. If possible, a sample should also be sent for culture.

Contra-indications to percutaneous biopsy are anticoagulation or coagulopathy, thrombocytopenia, and an FEV_1 of less than 1 l. Pneumothorax occurs in 20%, but is often asymptomatic and requires insertion of an intercostal tube in only 1% of all biopsies. Minor haemoptysis is common after the procedure, but is of sufficient severity to require intevention in only 1%.

Pleural aspiration/biopsy

1. Simple aspiration. Aspiration of pleural fluid is central to the investigation of pleural effusion. The site for aspiration is chosen taking account of the clinical signs and CXR appearances, or under ultrasound guidance. The skin and subcutaneous tissues are anaesthetized using 2% lignocaine with an orange (25G) needle. Blue (23G) and green (21G) needles are then used to anaesthetize the deeper layers. Applying gentle suction, a syringe with a white (19G) gauge needle is advanced until pleural fluid is obtained. If the tip of the needle comes up against a rib, the syringe should be withdrawn slightly and angled upwards to the interspace above before advancing again. When the pleural space is entered, fluid is withdrawn and sent for microscopy, culture, cytological examination and estimation of the protein content. Other measurements are discussed in the topic 'Pleural effusion'.

2. Abram's needle biopsy. Pleural biopsy in the presence of fluid is performed using an Abram's needle. It should not be performed in patients taking anticoagulants or with platelet counts of less than 50×10^9 per l. Two percent lignocaine is instilled as described for simple aspiration, and a sample of pleural fluid removed for analysis, if this has not been done previously. A stab incision is made using a number 11 blade, the depth of the incision being guided by the distance the needle had to be advanced in order to obtain pleural fluid during instillation of local anaesthetic. The Abram's trocar is then advanced in the closed position until the parietal pleura is penetrated. The trocar is then opened, rotated until the bevel is pointing downwards so that the intercostal neurovascular bundle is not damaged, pulled back until pleura is trapped in the bevel and then closed. On withdrawing the trochar, an assistant should hold a swab over the incision to prevent passage of air into the pleura. Six to ten biopsies should be taken, at least one being sent in saline for myobacterium tuberculosis (MTB) culture and the remainder in formalin for histology.

3. Tru-cut needle biopsy. A Tru-cut needle can be used to sample the pleura when it is so abnormal that it is over 1 cm in thickness. This technique can be performed in the absence of underlying pleural fluid. It is best used when there is generalized pleural thickening – more localized disease may necessitate ultrasound or radiographic screening for guidance. As with the Abram's needle, anticoagulation or coagulopathy are contra-indications. Tru-cut needles can also be used to obtain tissue samples from subcutaneous lumps and other lesions on the chest, and are especially useful when these are suspected of being metastatic malignant deposits.

Further reading

Toghill PJ. *Essential Medical Procedures*. London: Edward Arnold, 1997.

Related topics of interest

Fibre-optic bronchoscopy (p. 79)
Lung cancer (p. 97)
Pleural effusion (p. 117)
Thoracic surgical procedures (p. 154)

BREATHLESSNESS

The aetiology of the symptom of breathlessness is complex, involving the higher centres where breathlessness is perceived, the respiratory centres in the brainstem, carotid body, and receptors in the upper airway, lungs, articulations of the thoracic cage and the respiratory muscles. Current theories suggest that breathlessness is perceived when there is a discrepancy between the ventilation that the brain desires and that which is actually achieved.

Aetiology

This expected/achieved discrepancy can arise when the body's requirements for oxygen delivery and carbon dioxide elimination are normal, but there is impaired function of the heart, lungs or circulation.

1. Impaired ventilation. This may be caused by diseases of the airways (upper airway, asthma, chronic obstructive pulmonary disease (COPD)), lungs (fibrosis) or chest wall (scoliosis) which make it harder for the respiratory muscles to get air into the lungs, or by abnormalities of the muscles themselves.

2. Impaired oxygen transfer. The transfer of oxygen from air into the blood requires intact alveoli with pulmonary capillaries in close proximity. Abnormalities of the lungs (fibrosing alveolitis (FA)) or pulmonary circulation (pulmonary emboli, primary pulmonary hypertension) will impair this process.

3. Decreased transport. Oxygen passes from the lungs to the peripheral tissues as oxygenated haemoglobin. Anaemia or poor cardiac output reduce the amount of oxygen that is delivered to peripheral tissues.

There may also be an expected/achieved discrepancy when the lungs and heart are normal, if the expected ventilation is excessively high:

4. Stimulation of intra-pulmonary J receptors. This occurs in pneumonia, pulmonary embolism and pulmonary oedema.

5. Increased peripheral demand for oxygen. The metabolic demands of pregnancy and thyrotoxicosis require increased delivery of oxygen. Diseases of the joints or muscles often lead to recruitment of additional muscle groups for tasks such as walking, with the consequence that oxygen requirements are higher.

6. Increased chemical drive. Metabolic acidosis (e.g. diabetic ketoacidosis or salicylate poisoning) is a potent respiratory stimulant.

7. Psychogenic breathlessness. Hyperventilation syndromes and panic attacks involve the perception of the need for higher ventilation.

Clinical features

1. Onset. Sudden onset of breathlessness suggests diseases such as pulmonary embolism, pneumothorax, pulmonary oedema or pneumonia. A more insidious onset over a few months is more representative of malignancy or a pleural effusion. More chronic breathlessness suggests emphysema, COPD, pulmonary fibrosis or a myopathy. The breathlessness of asthma may follow any of these patterns.

2. Precipitating factors. Most patients complain that their breathlessness is worse on exercise, but other features may give a clue as to the cause. Exposure to allergens or dust may induce breathlessness. Nocturnal breathlessness is seen in left ventricular failure, asthma and diaphragmatic weakness. Immersion of the abdomen in water when entering a swimming pool or bath produces breathlessness in bilateral diaphragm paralysis. Orthopnoea is classically a feature of diaphragm paralysis or heart failure, but is also seen in many other diseases such as COPD. Platypnoea (breathlessness relieved by lying down) is more unusual: it suggests an atrial septal defect or arterio-venous malformations in the lower lobes, but is occasionally seen in FA. Breathlessness during episodes of anxiety or in stressful situations suggests hyperventilation.

3. Associated symptoms. Wheeze is a feature of asthma or COPD, but may also be described by patients with heart failure. Wheeze should be differentiated from the noise of stridor heard in upper airway obstruction. Excessive sighing and the feeling of being unable to take a full inspiration are features of psychogenic breathlessness, which may be associated with peripheral and peri-oral tingling.

Investigations

The baseline investigations required in a patient complaining of breathlessness are spirometry, CXR, haemoglobin, and an ECG. Other tests to consider thereafter are lung volumes, carbon monoxide transfer, arterial blood gases, ventilation–perfusion scan, echocardiogram and tests of respiratory muscle function. Home peak flow monitoring is valuable in patients with intermittent breathlessness who are suspected of having asthma. If the cause is still not apparent, a cardio-respiratory exercise test should be performed.

Management

The underlying condition causing breathlessness should be treated. Continuous oxygen via an oxygen concentrator is of value for patients who are hypoxic and breathless at rest, for example in severe FA Cylinders of oxygen can be of value if the patient desaturates on exercise, the smaller sizes being portable for travel outside the house. A cylinder of oxygen has a strong placebo effect, so objective documentation of desaturation, correctable by supplementary oxygen, should be obtained whenever possible.

In severe breathlessness benzodiazepines or opiates can be used. Non-invasive ventilation is an effective way of relieving orthopnoea in patients with neuromuscular disease. Breathing exercises and relaxation techniques can be of value in psychogenic breathlessness.

Further reading

Bourke SJ, Munro NC, White JES, *et al*. Platypnoea-orthodeoxia in cryptogenic fibrosing alveolitis. *Respiratory Medicine*, 1995; **89:** 387–389.

Davis CL. ABC of palliative care: breathlessness, cough and other respiratory problems. *British Medical Journal*, 1997; **315:** 931–934.

Lock SH, Paul EA, Rudd RM, Wedzicha JA. Portable oxygen therapy: assessment and usage. *Respiratory Medicine*, 1991; **85:** 407–412.

Toghill PJ. *Examining Patients*. London: Edward Arnold, 1995.

Related topics of interest

BRONCHIECTASIS

Bronchiectasis should really become a disease of the past, at least in developed countries, as a result of antibiotic treatment of childhood lower respiratory tract infections, immunization against pertussis (although the evidence for pertussis leading to bronchiectasis is weak), declining incidence of TB, intravenous immunoglobulin therapy in immunodeficiency, and the prospect of gene therapy for CF. That the condition is still an important clinical problem probably reflects the ease with which it can now be diagnosed using HRCT. Different anatomical subtypes are described in older textbooks (saccular, tubular, etc.), but these classifications are little used since the demise of bronchography.

Aetiology

1. Localized. Disease in the lower lobes, right middle lobe or lingula can follow a severe pneumonia, or obstruction of a bronchus by a foreign body (e.g. a peanut), tumour or extrinsic compression (e.g. tuberculous glands). Upper lobe bronchiectasis is usually caused by tuberculosis or allergic bronchopulmonary aspergillosis.

2. Generalized. Prolonged and recurrent lower respiratory tract infections associated with defects of immunity or mucociliary clearance lead to generalized bronchiectasis.

- CF.
- Ciliary dyskinetic syndromes, sometimes associated with situs inversus, sinusitis or infertility (e.g. in Young's and Kartagener's syndromes).
- Defects of humoral immunity such as hypogammaglobulinaemia almost invariably lead to bronchiectasis.
- Cartilage defects lead to dilation of bronchi (hence the term tracheobronchomegaly). These floppy airways tend to collapse prematurely during expiration and cough, impairing sputum clearance. Examples are the Williams Campbell and Mounier Kuhn syndromes.

Vasculitis and immune complex deposition probably underly the link between bronchiectasis and diseases such as rheumatoid arthritis (RA) and inflammatory bowel diseases. Rarer associations are alpha-1-antitrypsin deficiency, AIDS, Marfan's syndrome, Ehlers-Danlos syndrome, systemic lupus erythematosus (SLE), Sjogren's syndrome, sarcoidosis and the yellow nail syndrome.

Clinical features

The cough of bronchiectasis is usually productive of purulent sputum every day, with increasing purulence and volume during exacerbations. Haemoptysis occurs at some time in about 50% of cases, and is often recurrent. Shortness of breath and wheeze are features of more severe generalized bronchiectasis. In patients with mild disease there may be no clinical signs.

Coarse crackles, heard in early inspiration, are characteristic. These are also audible with the stethoscope held in front of the patient's mouth. Polyphonic expiratory wheezes are also common. Clubbing, cyanosis and cor pulmonale are seen in chronic severe generalized disease.

Investigations

Ring or tram-line shadows are seen on the CXR in 90% of patients with bronchiectasis. HRCT should be performed in patients with a clinical history suggestive of bronchiectasis in whom the CXR is normal, or when there is doubt about the cause of CXR shadowing. 'Signet-ring bronchi', thickened bronchi larger than their accompanying vessels, are characteristic on HRCT. Bronchiectasis confined to one or two lobes on a plain CXR often proves to be more widespread on HRCT.

Strep. pneumoniae and *H. influenzae* are the most common pathogens cultured from sputum, but colonization with *Pseudomonas* is also seen. Spirometry and home peak expiratory flow rate (PEFR) monitoring will identify airflow obstruction and assess variability. Arterial blood gases should be analysed in more severe disease with cyanosis and signs of cor pulmonale. Serum immunoglobulins (IgA, total IgG and sub-classes) and functional antibodies against *Strep. pneumoniae* and *H. influenzae* should be measured to identify immunodeficiency. The sweat test and other tests for CF are discussed under the topic 'Cystic Fibrosis'. The saccharin test is used as a screen for ciliary problems. This involves placing saccharin on the nasal mucosa through the anterior nares and waiting until a sweetness is tasted when the saccharin has been transported through the nose to reach the taste buds. Electron microscopy of nasal mucosal biopsy or radio-isotope mucus clearance studies are necessary for more precise documentation of ciliary defects.

Complications

Pneumonia in patients with bronchiectasis usually requires admission to hospital for treatment with physiotherapy, antibiotics and oxygen. Pneumothorax should always be considered as a cause of deteriorating breathlessness in patients with bronchiectasis. Massive haemoptysis occurs in less than 10% of cases, but can be life threatening and requires resection of a lobe. Cor pulmonale develops in the later stages of the disease. Amyloidosis in seen in chronic severe disease.

Management

Antibiotics for acute exacerbations, guided by sputum culture. Amoxycillin in conventional or high dose (3 g bd) can be used continuously to reduce the frequency of exacerbations. Quinolones are useful for pseudomonas colonization (e.g. ciprofloxacin 750 mg bd). Nebulized antiobiotics can also be used for prophylaxis, but are cumbersome to administer.

Bronchodilators, inhaled or nebulized, in patients with associated airflow obstruction. The response of airflow obstruction to steroids should be formally assessed during a period of clinical stability with Prednisolone 30 mg/day for 2 weeks.

Postural drainage should be performed daily. Huffing is valuable for expectoration, together with percussion if a suitable assistant is available at home. Skilled physiotherapy assistance helps with clearance of secretions during exacerbations. Intravenous immunoglobulin replacement can be given in hospital or at home for hypogammaglobulinaemia. Vaccination against pneumococcus and influenza is advisable. Mucolytics such as DNase are expensive and their place controversial.

Oxygen should be given for chronic hypoxia (PaO_2 <7.3 kPa on air) and cor pulmonale, as discussed in the topic 'chronic obstructive pulmonary disease'. Resection of affected lung is used for troublesome symptoms and localized disease in otherwise fit patients, or very rarely for massive threatening haemoptysis. Double lung or heart–lung transplantation should be considered in patients less than 60 years of age with an FEV_1 less than 30% predicted. If hypercapnic respiratory failure develops, non-invasive ventilation has been used as a bridge to transplantation.

Further reading

Van der Bruggen-Bogaarts BAHA, van der Bruggen HMJG, van Waes PFGM, Lammers J-WJ. Screening for bronchiectasis. *Chest* 1996; **109:** 608–611.

Related topics of interest

Aspergillus (p. 11)
Chronic obstructive pulmonary disease (p. 37)
Immunodeficiency (p. 90)
Mycobacteria (p. 105)
Pneumonia (p. 124)

CARDIAC DISORDERS

In the absence of a shunt, almost the entire cardiac output passes through the pulmonary circulation. The function of the lungs and the heart are thus intimately related. Some multisystem diseases, sarcoidosis or amyloidosis for example, may coincidentally involve the lungs and the heart. This topic will consider only those respiratory problems which are a direct consequence of abnormal cardiac function. Symptoms, signs, investigation and management of specific respiratory complications which are considered more fully in other topics will not be repeated here.

Clinical features

1. Acute heart failure. Pulmonary oedema occurs when left atrial pressure is elevated (mitral valve disease, left ventricular failure). The classical symptoms are orthopnoea and paroxysmal nocturnal dyspnoea, but these can be difficult to differentiate from the nocturnal symptoms of asthma and COPD, particularly if airway congestion in acute heart failure leads to wheeze. Radiographically, pulmonary oedema causes perihilar (bat's wing) shadowing, with Kerley B lines and bilateral pleural effusions. However, asymmetrical shadowing does occur. The differentiation of pulmonary oedema from pneumonia can be difficult, particularly in the elderly who may be apyrexial with pneumonia. It should be remembered that the two conditions can coexist if pneumonia precipitates heart failure or if heart failure becomes complicated by pneumonia.

2. Chronic heart failure. Differentiation of cardiac from pulmonary breathlessness may be difficult, for example in a smoker with both COPD and an ischaemic cardiomyopathy, and a cardio-respiratory exercise test may help distinguish between these two possibilities. Patients with chronic heart failure may have pleural effusions, usually transudates. Respiratory muscle weakness is well documented in chronic heart failure, but the contribution of this to symptoms is uncertain. Periodic respiration during sleep (Cheyne–Stokes) is associated with sleep disruption and daytime sleepiness; treatment with oxygen or nasal CPAP are effective.

3. Dressler's syndrome. Pleural effusion 4–6 weeks after acute myocardial infarction, associated with a high erythrocyte sedimentation rate (ESR) and pleuro-pericardial pain.

4. Emboli. Multiple lung abscesses are seen in right-sided endocarditis. Emboli may also be seen in atrial myxoma or other cardiac tumours.

5. Surgery. Cardiac surgery may cause respiratory complications, for example damage to the phrenic nerve.

6. Drugs. Several drugs used to treat cardiological conditions cause pulmonary complications (e.g. amiodarone).

Further reading

Chua TP, Coats AJS. The lungs in chronic heart failure. *European Heart Journal*, 1995; **16:** 882–887.

Related topics of interest

Drug-induced lung disease (p. 66)
Pleural effusion (p. 117)
Pneumonia (p. 124)

CHEST X-RAY

The CXR is an almost essential investigation in a patient with a respiratory problem. Comparison with old films is often valuable, and may save the patient unnecessary further investigation. Since X-rays are more commonly lost, mis-filed or destroyed than notes, it is good practice to draw a sketch of the CXR in the notes for future reference.

Views

The standard CXR is the postero-anterior (PA) film, taken on full inspiration. If this is diagnostic, for example of a pneumothorax, further imaging is unnecessary, but in most patients suspected of having a respiratory problem a lateral film should also be taken. If the patient is too unwell to attend the X-ray department, an antero-posterior film may be taken; departmental PA and lateral views should be obtained at the earliest opportunity. Films taken in expiration are commonly requested for patients suspected of having a pneumothorax, but are of no value in this setting: they may be useful to detect air trapping, for example in foreign body inhalation, McLeod's sydrome or a large bulla. CT scans have largely superseded apical or lordotic conventional CXRs, and ultrasound is superior to decubitus films in detecting pleural fluid.

Looking at the PA film

The CXR should be viewed systematically in all cases, to avoid the mistake of stopping after the first abnormality spotted. The following areas should be inspected in order:

1. Lung fields. The common types of lung shadowing are described below. Abnormal shadowing should be described as upper-, mid- or lower-zone, covering equal thirds of the lung fields. An abnormality in the upper zone may be in the apical segment of the lower lobe, and it is usually only possible to decide which lobe is abnormal after inspection of the lateral film. An exception to this is when there is an indication from the PA film as to how close a lesion is to a fixed anatomical structure; for example, shadowing in the right lower zone which obliterates the heart border must be in the right middle lobe, or a lesion in the left lower zone which leaves the heart border intact must be posterior and therefore in the left lower lobe.

2. Hilar regions. Hilar enlargement can be difficult to assess unless it is gross or very asymmetrical. The causes of a large hilum are either a mass such as a tumour or lymphadenopathy, or enlargement of the pulmonary arteries. In pulmonary hypertension the hilar shadow has a smooth outline and vessels can often clearly be seen emerging from the shadow, but CT will resolve any doubt.

3. Heart. The position of the heart gives important information about loss of volume and collapse (see below). Enlargement of the heart may suggest a cardiac cause for pleural effusions or lung shadowing.

4. Mediastinum. The remainder of the mediastinum should be examined, looking in particular for paratracheal lymphadenopathy, masses, a hiatus hernia, the dilated oesophagus of achalasia or a pharyngeal pouch. The causes of mediastinal masses and their anatomical distribution are described in the topic 'Developmental disorders and mediastinal disease'.

5. Diaphragms. The outline of the hemi-diaphragms should be smooth, with the right slightly higher than the left. Elevation of the hemi-diaphragm may be due to loss of lung volume in that hemithorax or paralysis of the muscle. Sub-pulmonary pleural effusions can mimic elevation of the hemi-diaphragm, but convexity of the shadow is more medial, and on the left side there may be a clue in the distance between the gastric air bubble and the apex of the 'diaphragm'. Obliteration of the costophrenic angle indicates pleural fluid or thickening. Loss of the diaphragmatic shadow is also seen when there is solid tissue adjacent to it (see below). Calcified plaques on the diaphragmatic pleura are characteristic of asbestos exposure.

6. Bones. Lytic or sclerotic lesions in the bones are usually due to malignancy. Exceptions include actinomycosis which invades through the pleura into bony structures.

7. Soft tissues. Finally, soft tissue abnormalities, sometimes evident on the PA film, are subcutaneous air, supra-clavicular masses, a mastectomy or breast implants.

Looking at the lateral film If a discrete lesion is seen on the PA film, the lateral film will usually facilitate more precise anatomical location. The relationship of shadowing to the horizontal and oblique fissures allows it to be placed in a particular lobe. Upper lobe shadowing leads to the anterior area behind the sternum above the heart being denser than normal. Lower lobe shadowing causes the lower thoracic vertebrae to be denser than normal. The appearances of collapse on the lateral CXR are described below.

Common abnormalities of the CXR *1. Consolidation.* The shadowing of consolidation may conform to a lobar or segmental distribution or be more patchy. Air bronchograms are characteristic.

2. Collapse. Occlusion of a bronchus leads to loss of volume or collapse of the lung distally. When this affects a main bronchus, the hemithorax on that side becomes opaque, with shift of the mediastinum towards that side.

Right upper lobe collapse causes shadowing in the upper zone with elevation of the horizontal fissure and deviation of the trachea to the right. Right middle lobe collapse causes blurring of the heart border on the PA film, with a characteristic triangular shadow between the horizontal and oblique fissures on the lateral view. Right lower lobe collapse causes movement of the heart to the right, with loss of the diaphragm shadow medially and a basal triangular shadow that does not obliterate the heart border; on the lateral view the vertebrae appear more opaque than normal inferiorly.

Left upper lobe collapse causes a haziness over the left mid- and upper-zones. Air in the apical segment of the left lower lobe clearly outlines the aortic arch; the trachea and heart may move to the left, and on the lateral view the oblique fissure is displaced anteriorly with opacification in front of it. Left lower lobe collapse leads to a white line adjacent to the left heart border, with opacification medial to this line and loss of the diaphragmatic shadow; the heart may move to the left, and on the lateral view the vertebrae appear more opaque than normal inferiorly.

3. Cavitation. This may be seen in a single lesion, or within a consolidated lobe. The differential diagnosis of cavitation is considered under the topic 'Pneumonia'.

4. Pleural effusion. The presence of fluid in the pleural cavity causes opacification with a concave upper border, unless the fluid is loculated. Air bronchograms are absent and, if large, the mediastinum is shifted away from the shadowing. Loculated pockets of air within a pleural effusion suggest an empyema of anaerobic aetiology. A straight horizontal surface to the effusion indicates the presence of air in addition to fluid in the pleural space.

5. Mass. The differential diagnosis of a mass lesion on the CXR is considered under the topic 'Lung cancer'.

6. Diffuse lung shadowing. The causes of diffuse opacities are listed under the topic 'Pneumoconiosis'.

7. Other abnormalities. Many other abnormalities may be seen on a CXR. Pneumothorax, pulmonary emboli, bronchiectasis, and arterio-venous malformations (AVM) are covered in their respective topics.

Further reading

Armstrong P, Wastie ML. *Diagnostic Imaging*. Oxford: Blackwell, 1998.
Corne J, Carroll M, Brown I, Delany D. *Chest X-ray Made Easy*. New York: Churchill Livingstone, 1997.

Related topics of interest

CHRONIC OBSTRUCTIVE PULMONARY DISEASE

COPD is a chronic progressive disease with fixed or poorly reversible airflow obstruction. Within the COPD population some patients will have predominant emphysema, and some may have undiagnosed chronic asthma in which airway remodelling has led to a substantial irreversible component to the airway obstruction.

Aetiology

COPD is caused by tobacco smoking (for causes of emphysema see the topic Emphysema).

Clinical features

The clinical features depend upon the severity of disease.

1. Mild COPD (FEV$_1$ 60–80% predicted). Patients will have minimal exertional dyspnoea and may have persistent cough. Examination is normal.

2. Moderate COPD (FEV$_1$ 40–59% predicted). Patients will have breathlessness on moderate exertion and may have a persistent cough. Examination may reveal early signs of lung hyperinflation, reduced air entry and wheeze.

3. Severe COPD (FEV$_1$ <40% predicted). Patients will have symptoms on minimal exertion or at rest with cough and wheeze. Examination will reveal signs of lung hyperinflation in addition to the signs present in moderate COPD. In addition in late, severe COPD patients may have evidence of respiratory failure (cyanosis) or cor pulmonale (signs of right heart failure).

Investigations

Spirometry will show a reduced FEV$_1$ to VC ratio. Severity can be categorized using the FEV$_1$ criteria listed above. Bronchodilator reversibility tests may be helpful in identifying chronic asthma; however many patients with COPD show some reversibility (typically 5–10%) with β_2 agonists or anticholinergic agents. The CXR may be normal or show hyperinflation. HRCT is useful in assessing the extent of emphysema or bullous disease if present, and should be reserved for individuals in whom surgery (bullectomy or lung volume reduction surgery (LVRS)) is being considered. Arterial blood gas measurements may be useful in patients with severe disease to assess the need for long-term oxygen therapy (LTOT).

Management

Guidelines are available on the management of patients with COPD in both the UK and the USA.

Maintenance treatment

- FEV$_1$ 80–100%: smoking cessation
- FEV$_1$ 60–80%: antibiotics for acute infections, as required bronchodilator (β_2 agonists)

- FEV$_1$ 40–59%: combination bronchodilators (β_2 agonists plus anticholinergic), steroid reversibility trial (see below), influenza vaccination
- FEV$_1$ 40%: as above plus assess for pulmonary rehabilitation, LTOT, nebulized bronchodilator therapy.

Steroid reversibility trials should be performed by measuring spirometry and/or serial peak flow before and after a 2-week course of prednisolone 30 mg. Twenty percent of patients show a significant (>15%) improvement. Theophyllines are of limited value in the routine management of COPD. Response to nebulized bronchodilator therapy for maintenance should be assessed using a formal trial as for steroids. About 20% of patients show significant (>15%) improvement in mean peak flow or FEV$_1$ but many more (50%) show subjective improvement in respiratory symptoms. Long-term oxygen therapy should be considered in patients with PaO$_2$ <7.3 kPa who increase their PaO$_2$ without a concomitant rise in PaCO$_2$ (>1 kPa).

Treatment of acute exacerbations

Mild exacerbations may be treated at home, with an increase in bronchodilator therapy and antibiotics if purulent sputum is present. A course of oral steroids should be given to patients who are steroid responsive or in whom reversibility to steroids has not been formally assessed if improvement is not seen with bronchodilators alone. Exacerbations failing to improve with the above measures may require hospitalization. Nebulized bronchodilators, intravenous aminophylline and oxygen in addition to the above measures should be used. Intermittent positive pressure ventilation (IPPV) may be appropriate when a reversible cause for the deterioration is present: however the decision to ventilate must be taken by an experienced doctor in consultation with the patient and family, and take into account the previous functional status. Nasal IPPV is an alternative approach which may be useful in those patients who can tolerate it during acute exacerbations.

Other treatments

Polycythaemia secondary to hypoxia may require venesection if the haematocrit is >0.55. Bullectomy may improve symptoms in individuals with a single large bulla surrounded by functional lung tissue. Rehabilitation programmes have been shown to produce short-term benefit in severe COPD.

LVRS involves removal of severely affected lung (usually by multiple wedge resections) and may improve symptoms, perhaps by increasing elastic recoil of the lung or by lowering FRC and thus aiding respiratory muscle function. LVRS should always be preceded by intensive pulmonary rehabilitation. In one large series, mortality was 4% and improvement in FEV_1 50% at 6 months. Criteria for LVRS are predominant emphysema, heterogeneity of parenchymal disease on HRCT, minimal co-morbidity and non-smokers.

Outcome Prognosis is dependent upon severity of the COPD presentation and rate of decline in FEV_1 which in turn is influenced by smoking cessation. Patients with severe COPD presenting with cor pulmonale have a poor prognosis (mean life expectancy 12–18 months).

Further reading

British Thoracic Society guidelines for the management of chronic obstructive pulmonary disease. *Thorax*, 1997; **53:** supplement 5.
Cooper JD *et al.* Results of 150 consecutive bilateral lung volume reduction procedures in patients with severe emphysema. *Journal of Thoracic and Cardiovascular Surgery*, 1996; **112:** 1319–1330.

Related topics of interest

CLINICAL EXAMINATION

Examination of a patient with a respiratory problem consists of a full assessment of the cardiovascular system, respiratory system and abdomen. The techniques involved for the respiratory system will be considered in this chapter. The degree of detail in which the nervous and musculoskeletal systems are examined will depend upon the particular clinical problem. Before embarking on this systematic examination, there are some more general clinical signs which are of particular relevance to the patient with a respiratory problem.

Hands

The causes of clubbing are listed below:

- Congenital.
- Bronchial carcinoma.
- FA, asbestosis.
- Chronic pulmonary sepsis (bronchiectasis, lung abscess).
- Infective endocarditis.
- Cyanotic congenital heart disease.
- Ulcerative colitis, Crohn's disease, cirrhosis, coeliac.
- Many other rare causes (e.g. pregnancy, arterio-venous (AV) malformations, lymphoma oesophageal problems (carcinoma/leiomyoma/achalasia), thymoma, thyroid carcinoma, leukaemia, atrial mxyoma).

Warm hands with a flapping tremor suggest carbon dioxide retention. Yellow nails are a rare association of chylothorax. Nicotine staining of the nails is a guide to the recent cigarette consumption. Wasting of the small muscles of the hand is seen with tumours at the apex of the lung invading the brachial plexus (Pancoast). The changes of scleroderma and rheumatoid arthritis (RA) may be apparent.

Eyes

Several ocular signs are relevant to the respiratory system (*Table 1*). Many of these will be revealed when then the eyes are examined fully as part of the nervous system, but some will be apparent during the preliminary general examination.

Neck

Swelling of the neck with distended non-pulsatile veins is seen in superior vena cava obstruction. Elevation of the jugular venous pressure is a sign of cor pulmonale, pulmonary embolism and pericardial constriction. Cervical lymphadenopathy raises the possibility of cancer, but lymphoma, tuberculosis and sarcoidosis should be borne in mind. A goitre may contribute to breathlessness or cause obstructive sleep apnoea (OSA). The scar of a phrenic nerve crush operation, performed before the introduction of anti-tuberculous chemotherapy, will invariably be associated with ipsilateral signs from pulmonary and pleural scarring. Subcutaneous emphysema indicates the presence of a pneumothorax.

Table 1.

Ocular manifestation	Respiratory association
Horner's syndrome	Pancoast tumour
Bilateral ptosis	Myaesthenia gravis
Proptosis	Wegener's granulomatosis
Conjunctivitis	Atopy
Cataracts	Long-term steroid usage
Uveitis	Sarcoidosis
Scleritis	Rheumatoid arthritis
	Wegener's granulomatosis
Jaundice	Metastatic carcinoma
	Pneumonia
	Cor pulmonale
Papilloedema	Hypercapnia
	Wegener's granulomatosis
	Sarcoidosis
Choroiditis	Tuberculosis
Retinal vasculitis	Systemic lupus erythematosus
Retinopathy	Carcinoma, human immuno-deficiency virus
Keratoconjunctivitis	Sjogren's syndrome
Orbital oedema	Superior vena cava obstruction
Surgical emphysema	Pneumothorax

Mouth

Oral manifestations and associations of respiratory diseases are listed in *Table 2*.

Assessment of the mouth is also important in patients with OSA, looking for tonsillar enlargement, macroglossia and retrognathia.

Skin

Non-dermatologists are often guilty of looking through the skin rather than at it, but full examination of this organ can give valuable clues about underlying respiratory disease (*Table 3*).

Chest

1. Inspection. Scars of previous surgery or intercostal drains may be apparent. Obesity or thoracic deformities such as pectus excavatum, kyphosis or scoliosis may cause or contribute to breathlessness. COPD is suggested by a barrel-shaped chest. Collapse of an upper lobe may result in visible depression of the upper ribcage, when compared with the contralateral side.

A fast respiratory rate is a feature of many respiratory diseases, but attention should be paid to the relative times spent in inspiration and expiration which may give a clue as to whether the problem is related to airway obstruction, in which case expiration is prolonged. Pursed-lip breathing also suggests severe COPD.

Table 2.

Oral manifestation	Respiratory association
Poor dentition	Lung abscess
Periodontitis	Actinomycosis
Missing tooth	Inhalation
Ulceration	Herpes simplex in immunodeficiency
	Tuberculosis
	Behcet's syndrome
	Wegener's granulomatosis, SLE
Herpetic stomatitis	Pneumonia
	Immunodeficiency
Kaposi's sarcoma	Acquired immunodeficiency syndrome
Candidiasis	Inhaled steroids
	Immunodeficiency
Parotitis	Sarcoidosis, tuberculosis, actinomycosis
Microstomia	Systemic sclerosis
Xerostomia	Sjogren's syndrome
Telangiectasis	Pulmonary AV malformations
Erythema multiforme	Pneumonia
Central cyanosis	Hypoxaemia

Table 3.

Dermatological condition	Respiratory association
Metastases	Cancer
Acanthosis nigricans	Cancer
Lupus pernio	Sarcoidosis
Cutaneous nodules	Sarcoidosis
Erythema nodosum	Sarcoidosis, tuberculosis
Lupus erythematosus	SLE
Erythema multiforme	Pneumonia (mycoplasma)
Lupus vulgaris	Tuberculosis
Telangectasis	Systemic sclerosis, Pulmonary arteriovenous malformations
Eczema	Asthma
Gynaecomastia	Cancer
Bruising	Long-term steroid usage

The pattern of movement of the chest also gives important diagnostic clues. Paradoxical inward motion of the lower ribcage during inspiration (Hoover's sign) is seen in patients with severe COPD, when the lungs are over-inflated and the diaphragm flat. Paradoxical inward motion of the abdomen during inspiration, often best seen with the patient lying supine, is a sign of bilateral diaphragm weakness. Paradoxical inward motion of the ribcage during inspiration is seen when the intercostal muscles are paralysed but diaphragmatic function is well preserved. Respiratory alternans, with alternate breaths being taken using the ribcage and abdominal compartments of the thoracic cage, is sometimes seen in patients with severe respiratory failure.

Accessory muscle recruitment is a non-specific sign of respiratory distress. Kussmaul's respiration describes the 'air hunger' of acidosis. Cheyne–Stokes or 'periodic' respiration is common during sleep or in patients with impaired consciousness. In an awake patient it suggests severe heart failure.

2. Palpation. Subcutaneous emphysema indicates the presence of a pneumothorax. Palpation of the trachea and apex beat will determine the position of the mediastinum. A right ventricular heave indicates chronic pulmonary hypertension.

Expansion of the chest should be assessed by placing the hands on the front of the upper part of the ribcage and noting the anterior motion of the ribcage when the patient takes a deep breath in. The hands are then placed around the sides of the lower ribcage and the lateral motion during a deep breath in noted. Posteriorly assessment of expansion should be limited to the lower ribcage, as even in normal subjects there is little motion of the upper ribcage posteriorly. Asymmetrical expansion of the ribcage has a number of causes (occlusion of bronchus, consolidation, fibrosis, pleural disease), differentiation of which requires percussion and auscultation.

3. Percussion. Percussion should begin below the clavicles and continue along a line over the anterior ribcage extending laterally into the axilla. Percussion should be performed in approximately four positions along this line on each side. A similar number of sites should be tested posteriorly, commencing medial to the scapula superiorly but moving more laterally lower down.

Hyper-resonance suggests a pneumothorax, bulla or herniation of gas-filled bowel into the chest. The percussion note is dull over pneumonia, pleural fluid, solid tissue (such as a large tumour), and the liver.

4. Auscultation. Auscultation should begin by listening to breathing without the aid of a stethoscope to detect stridor in patients with upper airway obstruction. The stethoscope should then be placed in similar sites to those described for percussion.

Breath sounds may be normal, reduced or increased; 'vesicular breath sounds' and 'normal air entry' are commonly used terms which should be avoided. Increased breath sounds (bronchial breathing) suggest consolidation or fibrosis. Decreased breath sounds can be caused by occlusion of a bronchus, or interposition of air or fluid between the lung and the stethoscope.

Added sounds, such as wheezes and crackles, should be described fully as to their timing (late inspiratory, early inspiratory) and character (monophonic, polyphonic). Fine inspiratory crackles are often heard at the lung bases during the first few deep breaths in a bed-bound patient. These are probably caused by re-expansion of atelectatic lung. Pathological crackles persist after these initial breaths. Coarse crackles caused by secretions in the large airways should clear on coughing. Crackles originating in the airways are characteristically coarse and early inspiratory. They may be audible at the mouth. Alveolar crackles are fine and pan- or late-inspiratory in timing.

A monophonic wheeze suggests narrowing of a single main bronchus. Polyphonic wheezes are heard in diffuse airway diseases. Mid-inspiratory squeaks are heard in bronchiolitis, particularly extrinsic allergic bronchiolo-alveolitis.

Other abnormal sounds on auscultation are a pleural rub, bruits over an AVM, a click in time with cardiac systole with a left-sided pneumothorax and bowel sounds when the diaphragm is elevated.

Cardiovascular system

On examination of the cardiovascular system, cor pulmonale may be apparent. Left heart failure may explain the presence of basal crackles or a pleural effusion. Right-sided endocarditis can lead to septic emboli to the lungs. A right-to-left intracardiac shunt may be the cause of arterial hypoxaemia.

Abdomen

Hepatomegaly occurs in right heart failure, secondary deposits from a bronchial carcinoma, some causes of cirrhosis or a hepatic abscess (leading to an empyema). Splenomegaly may be seen in sarcoidosis and TB. Ascites may be associated with pleural effusions.

Nervous system

Proximal myopathy is associated with steroids, respiratory muscle weakness, or as a paraneoplastic effect of lung cancer. Peripheral neuropathy may be caused by chronic hypoxaemia, or a paraneoplastic syndrome. Delirium may be the presenting feature of many respiratory diseases associated with either derangement of arterial blood gases, hypercalcaemia or inappropriate anti-diuretic hormone secretion. Cerebellar signs may indicate a paraneoplastic syndrome, or secondaries from a carcinoma. Other focal neurological defects may be caused by cerebral metastases or spinal cord compression.

Musculoskeletal system Several arthritides are associated with respiratory disease (see 'Rheumatological disorders').

Further reading

Forgacs P. *Lung Sounds*. London: Baillière Tindall, 1979.
Toghill PJ. *Examining Patients*. London: Edward Arnold, 1995.

Related topics of interest

Cardiac disorders (p. 28)
Clinical history (p. 46)
Digestive tract disorders (p. 64)
Neuromuscular disorders (p. 111)
Rheumatological disorders (p. 144)
Skeletal disorders (p. 150)

CLINICAL HISTORY

Respiratory symptoms have many different causes but taking a careful and detailed history from the patient will usually shorten the list of possible diagnoses to a handful. The commonest symptoms of respiratory diseases are covered in separate topics (see 'Breathlessness', 'Cough' and 'Haemoptysis'). In a patient who may have a respiratory disease, particular attention should be paid to the following aspects of the clinical history.

Smoking

Smoking is an important cause of respiratory disease in the developed world. Patients frequently deny being a smoker, although they may have only stopped smoking the previous week when they started to cough up blood. They should be asked the age at which they started to smoke and the average number of cigarettes smoked per day. Dividing the average intake by 20 and multiplying by the number of years they have smoked gives the 'pack-years' for that individual. Passive smoking in the home or workplace may be of relevance in a patient who complains of a chronic cough.

Occupation

In patients suspected of having respiratory disease related to an occupational exposure, the history should cover not only the patient's current job, but all occupations since leaving school. The exact nature of the job should be explored, documenting the particular dusts or fumes which may have been inhaled. The relationship of respiratory symptoms to the work pattern should be explored, for example the 'Monday morning fever' of a welder or whether symptoms improve at weekends or during holidays, as in occupational asthma. Many patients may be unaware, however, that they are likely to have been exposed to a substance which may be of relevance to their lung disease, for example asbestos in the construction industry or isocyanates in welders. Sometimes the occupation of another member of the family may be relevant, for example asbestos dust brought home on a man's overalls may be implicated as the cause of his wife's mesothelioma.

Pets

Pets are a common source of allergen, and can also be the origin of infections such as Chlamydia psittacii. Problems with birds are not confined to the owners, allergic alveolitis sometimes being caused by aviaries or pigeon lofts in neighbouring gardens.

Hobbies

Hobbies may centre round pets: horses or pigeons for example. Bronchoconstriction can be caused by the sulphurous fumes from sterilization of home brewing equipment, or soldering using colophony. A glance around any DIY store will show the wide range of chemicals which a patient may be exposed to, many of which could contribute to respiratory symptoms, particularly asthma.

Travel

Recent foreign travel adds to the spectrum of agents to be considered in pulmonary infections. Antibiotic resistance varies in different parts of the world, particularly in tuberculous or pneumococcal infection, and the areas visited may influence the choice of antibiotic. Sedentary periods during long journeys are a recognized risk factor for deep venous thrombosis and pulmonary embolism.

Drugs

The history should include a full list of drugs, both prescribed and over-the-counter remedies. Many patients do not regard agents such as aspirin, liquid paraffin, or indeed inhalers as 'drugs'. The use of 'alternative' medicines should be enquired about, and also recreational drugs.

Risk factors for HIV

In a patient with a respiratory infection which could be opportunistic, the patient should be asked about blood transfusions, intra-venous drug abuse and sexual contact which might predispose to HIV infection.

The family

Asthma, eczema and allergic rhinitis in the family suggest a genetic predisposition to asthma. A family history of emphysema may point to the diagnosis of alpha-1-antitrypsin or other protease deficiency. Patients are likely to have acquired TB if, when a child, another household member had the disease. Reactivation may occur in later life to cause overt disease.

Past medical history

Recurrent childhood infections raise the possibility of underlying immunodeficiency, or leave permanent damage, as in bronchiectasis. Alternatively, such 'infections' may have been asthma which was mis-diagnosed. Many older patients report having regular CXR for shadows on the lung when they were younger, suggesting infection with TB. This may be of relevance to the investigation of an abnormal CXR later in life. If the patient has had previous surgical procedures, it is worth enquiring about difficulties in recovery from anaesthesia or admission to an intensive care unit post-operatively, which may indicate poor respiratory reserve, such as a latent neuro-muscular problem.

Many systemic diseases have associated respiratory complications. A history of a particular systemic disease should prompt enquiry about symptoms of the relevant respiratory associations. Conversely, if the respiratory symptoms suggest a particular condition, the patient should be asked about symptoms of the systemic diseases which are associated with this condition.

Further reading

Toghill PJ. *Examining Patients*. London: Edward Arnold, 1995.

Related topics of interest

Breathlessness (p. 25)
Clinical examination (p. 40)
Cough (p. 49)
Haemoptysis (p. 83)

COUGH

Cough receptors are widely distributed throughout the upper and lower respiratory tracts, and this symptom can be associated with many different diseases. In around 10% of patients with a chronic cough no cause is found.

Aetiology

1. Acute. Viral upper respiratory tract infections are the commonest cause of cough, but the illness is usually self-limiting and does not require further investigation. Cough is also a prominent symptom in infective exacerbations of COPD and pneumonia.

2. Chronic. Common causes of cough lasting for more than 2 weeks are as follows:

- Asthma.
- COPD.
- Oesophageal reflux.
- Nasal pathology (post-nasal drip)/sinusitis.
- Bronchiectasis.
- Lung cancer.
- Tuberculosis.
- Cardiac failure.
- Pulmonary fibrosis.
- Pulmonary emboli.
- Inhaled foreign body.
- Angiotensin converting enzyme inhibitors.

Clinical features

1. Onset and duration. An acute febrile illness with a cough productive of purulent sputum suggests bronchitis, tracheitis or pneumonia; persistance of a cough productive of discoloured and foul-tasting sputum for more than a few days suggests the development of a lung abscess. A cough of longer duration is unlikely to have a simple infective aetiology.

2. Precipitating factors. Cough on exercise can be a pointer to asthma, even in the absence of wheeze; nocturnal or early morning cough is also characteristic of this disease, and there may be a seasonal pattern or association with allergen exposure. Cough on swallowing points to pharyngeal or laryngeal problems leading to aspiration – patients sometimes report a cough which has persisted since an acute episode of choking on food, when a pea or other food was inhaled. Cough on lying down is seen with oesophageal reflux and spill-over of gastric contents onto the larynx. Nasal blockage, sneezing and sensation of catarrh in the throat suggest rhinosinusitis and post-nasal drip as the cause of cough.

3. Associated symptoms. Haemoptysis is a pointer to the presence of a lung cancer, but is seen in many other conditions.

Weight loss in association with cough also increases the likelihood of a malignant aetiology, but could also be explained by TB. Chronic sputum production raises the possibility of COPD or bronchiectasis. Large volumes of sputum (bronchorrhoea) point to alveolar cell carcinoma. Inhaled food substances may be recognizable in the sputum. Shortness of breath occurs with cough caused by airway (asthma, COPD) or parenchymal lung disease (FA, EAA), but cough may be the dominant symptom in any of these conditions.

Investigations

If cough persists for more than 2 weeks, most patients will require a CXR. If a pulmonary cause is not seen, there are no worrying features in the history to suggest malignancy (e.g. haemoptysis, weight loss) and the heart size is normal, spirometry and home peak flow monitoring should be performed. If there is any suggestion of variable airflow obstruction, it may be appropriate to proceed to a therapeutic trial of bronchodilators or oral prednisolone. Other common diagnoses to consider at this stage are rhinosinusitis and gastro-oesophageal reflux. Oesophageal pH monitoring can be performed, but it is simpler to undertake a trial of anti-reflux therapy.

If the cause is still not apparent and the cough persists, bronchoscopy should be performed to look for a tumour or foreign body; this examination is also useful to exclude for laryngeal pathology as the cause of cough. Flow-volume loops can be performed prior to bronchoscopy, to look for an upper airway problem. Subsequently it may be necessary to proceed to provocation tests such as methacholine challenge or exercise. High resolution CT scanning of the chest is indicated if the clinical history points to bronchiectasis, since the CXR is normal in 10% of patients with this disease.

Management

In most patients, cough will subside with treatment of the underlying condition. Persistent unexplained cough is resistant to treatment. Nebulized therapy with local anaesthetics or opiates has proven disappointing, and oral opiates are often the only effective cough suppressant.

Further reading

Davis CL. ABC of palliative care: breathlessness, cough and other respiratory problems. *British Medical Journal*, 1997; **315:** 931–934.

Thidens HA, de Bock GH, Dekker FW, *et al*. Identifying asthma and chronic obstructive pulmonary disease in patients with persistent cough presenting to general practitioners: descriptive study. *British Medical Journal*, 1998; **316:** 1286–1290.

Toghill PJ. *Examining Patients*. London: Edward Arnold, 1995.

Related topics of interest

CYSTIC FIBROSIS

CF is the most important inherited lung disease. However, not all patients present with respiratory systems; some present in the neonatal period with meconium ileus and others in early childhood with failure to thrive or malabsorption. This topic deals with the respiratory complications of CF.

The incidence of CF is about 1 in 4000 live births in the UK. The inheritance of CF follows a classical Mendelian autosomal recessive genetic pattern. The carrier rate for the gene is 1 in 30; therefore the risk of two carriers becoming parents is, in theory, 1 in 900, and the likelihood of an affected individual being born to those parents is 1 in 900 $\times$ 4, that is 1 in 3600. In practice the actual incidence of affected births is slightly lower due to the influence of genetic counselling and deaths *in utero*. The high carrier rate for the mutation implies a selection advantage for heterozygotes: the explanation remains uncertain, although it has been suggested that heterozygotes have in the past been partially protected from severe secretory diarrhoea, for example due to cholera.

Aetiology

The clinical features of CF are due to a defect in membrane ion transport. The CF gene (on chromosome 7) has been cloned; the gene product is known as CFTR (CF transmembrane (conductance) regulator). This functions as a chloride channel in the apical cell membrane. Affected individuals have a non-functional channel owing to mutations within the CFTR gene and hence have abnormal chloride and, therefore, solute transport across secretory epithelia. In the lungs this results in increased mucus viscosity which, in turn, increases the likelihood of bacterial infection. DNA released from bacteria in the airways also increases mucus viscosity. Recurrent infections lead to the widespread bronchiectasis which is the hallmark of the disease and which ultimately leads to respiratory failure. Seventy percent of affected individuals in Europe carry the ΔF508 mutation; however, over 500 other mutations have been described, some of which result in at least some functional CFTR protein being produced. There is a relatively weak correlation between disease phenotype and the particular mutation present. In addition to a defect in chloride transport a second defect in sodium transport is evident in affected individuals with decreased sodium reabsorption across secretory epithelia. Whether or not this is due to a second associated defect in a sodium channel or is purely a paraphenomenon related to the defect in chloride transport remains uncertain. This may also be important in that altered airway lining fluid [Na^+] may inhibit defensin activity (defensins are constitutively expressed antimicrobial peptides).

Clinical features

Patients with meconium ileus (10–20%) present at birth. The majority of patients with respiratory disease present with recurrent chest infections during the first 10 years of life.

Occasional patients, particularly those with less severe mutations, present with bronchiectasis or recurrent chest infections later in life. Airway hyperreactivity is a common finding in CF.

The typical patient with advanced disease is thin owing to the combination of the increased metabolic rate (resulting from infection, increased workload owing to respiratory compromise, and malabsorption owing to pancreatic dysfunction). On auscultation widespread crackles owing to bronchiectasis are evident. Patients in respiratory failure will be cyanosed and are frequently clubbed and may have evidence of right ventricular hypertrophy, pulmonary hypertension and, in the late stages of disease, right heart failure.

Cholelithiasis (10–15%) and biliary cirrhosis (<5%) may occur. Infertility affects 95% of males and 20% of females with CF.

Investigations

The diagnosis used to be made by measuring sodium concentrations in sweat (>50 mmol/l being diagnostic). However, PCR-based diagnosis, either on a blood sample or using cheek cells, is the diagnostic test of choice where available and when the mutation is known: PCR can also be used for prenatal diagnosis. In the UK most PCR screening is designed to detect the three commonest mutations, which identify more than 90% of affected individuals.

The CXR may show evidence of bronchiectasis: this is almost invariably widespread throughout both lungs in later stages of CF. Patients with CF have a progressive decline in lung function. FEV_1 and VC are useful for monitoring disease progression.

Management

Patients with CF should be managed in recognized centres experienced in the care of this group of patients with the necessary support from a multidisciplinary team. Intensive treatment should be given to deal rapidly with infection. Survival trends over recent years have shown this approach improves the long-term outcome. When stable, patients should perform daily chest physiotherapy at home to help aid sputum clearance.

1. Infection. Infection should be dealt with promptly by appropriate antibiotics depending on the sensitivity of the organism. Initially colonization with organisms such as *H. influenzae* and *Staph. aureus* occurs, but many patients become infected with resistant organisms which may be difficult to treat. *Pseudomonas aeruginosa* and *Burkholderia cepacia* infection are particular problems requiring courses of either intravenous or nebulized antibiotics, although resistance is common. Patients with advanced disease may need long-term venous access via a tunnelled line for antibiotic treatment. Avoidance of cross-infection is important in preventing the spread of resistant organisms.

2. *Bronchodilators.* Many patients with CF respond to bronchodilator therapy, either inhaled or, in more advanced disease, via a nebulizer.

3. *Malabsorption.* Pancreatic insufficiency leading to malabsorption of fat and protein is present from birth in most patients with CF. Pancreatic enzyme (plus fat-soluble vitamin) supplements are necessary for the majority of patients with moderate or severe disease.

4. *Recombinant DNase.* The rationale for administering DNase is that the presence of bacterial DNA increases sputum viscosity. Trials with recombinant DNase show possible therapeutic benefit although at present this is not standard therapy.

5. *Lung transplantation.* This usually requires heart–lung transplantation owing to the pulmonary hypertension and right ventricular hypertrophy which accompany severe disease, potentially offering both symptomatic and prognostic benefits for patients with CF. However, the experience in general has been disappointing compared with other conditions for which transplantation has been used. This is probably due to the increased risk of the procedure in patients with chronic respiratory infection who subsequently need to be immunosuppressed.

6. *Gene therapy.* Preliminary gene therapy trials have established that the CFTR gene can be administered to the upper airways and expression achieved in respiratory epithelium. However, the levels of expression have been insufficiently high to produce a marked clinical effect. Two forms of administering the CFTR gene have been used: liposomal transfection and adenovirus-mediated transfection. The latter has the potential difficulty that an immune response may be mounted to repeated administration of the adenovirus vector. However, in the long term gene therapy offers a potential cure for the disease.

Outcome

The mean survival for patients with CF has increased by 50% from 1971 to 1990. This improvement is entirely due to intensive treatment, particularly for respiratory infection. Patients usually die as a consequence of respiratory failure.

Further reading

Davidson DJ, Porteous DJ. The genetics of cystic fibrosis lung disease. *Thorax*, 1998; **53:** 389–397.

Related topic of interest

Bronchiectasis (p. 28)

DEVELOPMENTAL DISORDERS AND MEDIASTINAL DISEASE

Mediastinal disease

The most frequently encountered mediastinal disorders are as follows:

- Primary tumour arising in mediastinum.
- Metastatic tumour (especially lymph node).
- Other causes of lymphadenopathy (e.g. sarcoidosis, TB).
- Mediastinitis: chemical (e.g. due to oesophageal perforation).
- Mediastinitis: inflammatory (e.g. due to drugs).
- Pneumomediastinum.
- Retrosternal goitre.
- Developmental cysts.
- Vascular abnormalities.
- Pericardial disease (effusions, cysts, constrictive pericarditis).

Clinical features

With the exception of mediastinitis which presents with pain and fever, presentation of mediastinal disease depends on the involvement of specific mediastinal structures. For practical purposes the structural abnormalities in the mediastinum can be grouped into anterior mediastinal masses (e.g. thymoma), posterior mediastinal lesions (e.g. neurofibroma) and other mediastinal disease (tumour, lymphadenopathy). Mediastinal masses may be asymptomatic or cause symptoms from local pressure: anterior and posterior mediastinal masses are likely to present as chance findings on an X-ray whereas mediastinal disease which compresses the oesophagus (producing dysphagia), the trachea (causing stridor), lymphatic drainage (causing pleural effusion) or the superior vena cava (SVC – causing obstruction) will present with symptoms resulting from local effects.

Malignancy

The most frequently seen primary tumours arising from within the mediastinum are oesophageal in origin, although many other rare tumours can arise from other elements from within the mediastinum. Malignant mediastinal lymphadenopathy is most frequently seen in the context of bronchial carcinoma but may occur with almost any tumour. Lymphoma frequently presents with mediastinal lymph node masses which may also cause large unilateral pleural effusions owing to obstruction of lymphatic drainage.

Thymoma

Tumours arising from the thymic remnant produce an anterior mediastinal mass on CXR. These may present with local obstruction (e.g. SVC), pleural or pericardial effusions or myasthenia gravis owing to the associated circulating antibodies directed against the acetylcholine receptor. Treatment is resection because of the potential for malignant transformation. Malignant thymoma may be amenable to surgery, or a chemotherapeutic approach.

Other tumours and cysts Congenital abnormalities arising from either the bronchus or the foregut occur in the mediastinum usually on the right side. These are usually asymptomatic but may present with infection or rupture. Many other rare primary tumours may arise in the mediastinum: the most frequent of these are from neural elements (e.g. neurofibroma, neuroblastoma), teratomas, and connective tissue tumours such as fibrosarcoma, lipomas, and haemangiomas. The mediastinum may also be involved in mesothelioma.

Mediastinal fibrosis A non-malignant but progressive fibrotic process can occur in the mediastinum: the features are similar to those seen in retroperitoneal fibrosis with local symptoms resulting from fibrosis. The aetiology is often unclear but in some cases drugs such as practolol have been implicated.

Vascular abnormalities Thoracic aortic aneurysms or rarely aneurysms in other vessels within the mediastinum may present as apparent mediastinal masses. CT scanning with contrast or MR angiography will confirm the diagnosis.

Pericardial disease Developmental cysts arising from the pericardium can present as apparent mediastinal masses on CXR. The pericardium can also be involved by malignancy, TB or connective tissue diseases (e.g. RA) resulting in pericardial effusions or constrictive pericarditis.

Developmental disorders

Bronchogenic cysts These are congenital abnormalities: they are commonest on the right side at the tracheo-bronchial junction. Bronchogenic cysts are usually asymptomatic but may present with symptoms resulting from local infection, haemoptysis, or rupture.

Pulmonary sequestration This occurs when a segment of lung has an aberrant blood supply and an anatomical defect in the bronchial system and usually presents with recurrent infection and/or an abnormal CXR. CT with contrast may help in the diagnosis. Surgical removal may be necessary for recurrent infection.

Diaphragmatic hernias Congenital diaphragmatic herniae are classified as anterior (Morgagni) or posterior (Bochdalek). The latter are more common (90%) and usually occur on the left. They may cause respiratory compromise and require surgical repair. Morgagni herniae have narrower necks and carry a higher risk of bowel strangulation.

In adulthood, diaphragmatic eventration is often an asymptomatic finding on the CXR, which can be difficult to differentiate from diaphragmatic paralysis. However, close inspection of the PA and lateral CXR often reveals that the elevation does not involve the whole hemi-diaphragm but is localized to one part of it. Respiratory compromise is extremely unusual and surgical intervention rarely necessary.

McCleod's syndrome

This is believed to arise because of abnormal development of one lung resulting in a hyperlucent hemithorax on CXR owing to a hypoplastic lung.

Arterio-venous malformations

Pulmonary AVMs may present with an abnormal CXR, or with haemoptysis. Patients with hereditary haemorrhagic telangiectasis (Osler–Weber–Rendu syndrome) are at markedly increased risk of AVMs, which are commonest in the lungs, brain and liver. This condition is inherited as an autosomal dominant disorder: at least three genetic loci have been identified. The diagnosis may be confirmed by angiography, CT with contrast, or MR angiography. There is an argument to embolize (or resect) AVMs because of the risk of paradoxical emboli (30% over 10 years) and massive haemoptysis; however, recurrence is common. Some patients present with exertional breathlessness and hypoxia owing to the magnitude of the shunt.

Further reading

Mole TM, Glover J, Shepperd MN. Sclerosing mediastinitis: a report on 18 cases. *Thorax*, 1995; **50:** 280–283.

Davis RD, Oldham HN, Sabiston DC. Primary cysts and neoplasms of the mediastinum: recent changes in clinical presentation, methods of diagnosis, management and results. *Annals of Thoracic Surgery*, 1987; **44:** 229–238.

Clements BS, Warner JO. Pulmonary sequestration and related bronchopulmonary-vascular malformations: nomenclature and classification based on anatomical and embryological considerations. *Thorax*, 1987; **42:** 401–408.

Gassage JR, Kanj G. Pulmonary arteriovenous malformations. *American Journal of Respiratory Critical Care Medicine*, 1998; **158:** 643–661.

Related topics of interest

DIFFUSE PARENCHYMAL LUNG DISEASE

Diffuse parenchymal lung disease (DPLD) has replaced terms such as insterstitial lung disease and pulmonary fibrosis.

Cryptogenic fibrosing alveolitis

Annual mortality from CFA in England and Wales has increased threefold since the early 1980s to about 1000 deaths per year currently. Mortality is increasing in both sexes, particularly in the elderly. Similar trends are seen in Australia. The current prevalence in the UK is up to 20 in 100 000, with a 2:1 male:female ratio. Median age at presentation is 67 years.

1. Aetiology. CFA is probably initiated by many different agents. The male predominance and similarity with asbestosis suggest occupational exposures may be important. Metal and wood dusts may be responsible for about 20% of cases. The acute onset in some patients, and the occasional FA arising after specific infections, suggests infection may play a role. There is an association with antidepressant use. There is no convincing histocompatibility leukocyte antigen (HLA) association.

Histologically, there is a mixed cellular infiltrate (lymphocytes, plasma cells) with fibroblast proliferation and collagen in alveolar walls. It is likely that initial inflammation precedes fibrosis. However, the disease is patchy, and areas of both cellular infiltration and fibrosis can be found in the same biopsy specimen.

2. Clinical features. The British Thoracic Society study reported in 1997 on nearly 600 patients with CFA. At presentation, patients have been symptomatic for a mean of 15 months. Almost all patients present with breathlessness, but 5% are initially asymptomatic. In 80% the onset of breathlessness is gradual, but in others the illness appears to begin with an acute respiratory infection. Cough (75%) and arthralgia (19%) are other features. Clubbing occurs in about 50%. Bibasal late inspiratory crackles, like 'unzipping velcro' are typical. Expiratory crackles, cyanosis and cor pulmonale are late features.

3. Investigations. Blood tests are unhelpful diagnostically. A mildly elevated ESR is common, and low titre antinuclear or rheumatoid factors are present in about 25%. Lung function tests show a restrictive defect with reduced gas transfer. CXR shows reticulonodular shadowing, predominantly lower zone and peripheral, and reduction in lung size. Pleural shadowing suggests other diagnoses. The lung shadowing often extends to other zones, and honeycombing may develop. HRCT shows a characteristic sub-pleural pattern of reticular and ground glass opacification, initially basal but becoming more extensive.

4. Diagnosis. A clinical diagnosis of CFA can be made in a patient with typical crackles, CXR and HRCT, restrictive lung function and no history of exposure to fibrogenic agents. Clubbing is supportive.

The need for biopsy has been debated because the reliability of a clinical diagnosis is unknown. Biopsy should be strongly considered in younger patients (in whom more unusual diagnoses may occur), or when there are unusual clinical or HRCT features. Transbronchial biopsy is unreliable for the diagnosis of CFA because of small sample size, and a surgical biopsy is required.

5. Management. Steroids are the most common treatment, but have never been subject to a placebo-controlled trial. Prednisolone is usually started at 0.5 mg/kg daily. Symptomatic improvement is seen in about 50% patients, but in lung function in only 25%. Any steroid response usually occurs in the first 1–2 months. In non-responders, prednisolone should be withdrawn over about 1 month, to avoid steroid side-effects. In responders, prednisolone is tapered over 6 months to a daily maintenance dose of about 10 mg.

Both cyclophosphamide and azathioprine have been evaluated in combination with prednisolone, versus prednisolone alone. No significant benefit was found with cyclophosphamide. Azathioprine was associated with significantly improved survival (57% versus 23% at 9 years for azathioprine and prednisolone as against prednisolone alone) and a low toxicity. Combined therapy with prednisolone and azathioprine (2–3 mg/kg) may be the best option. Colchicine may be as effective as prednisolone with fewer side effects.

In late disease with cor pulmonale diuretics are often needed, and domiciliary oxygen using a concentrator for severely breathless hypoxic patients. Younger patients with severe disease, not responding to treatment, should be considered for single lung transplantation.

6. Outcome. The course of CFA varies widely, from steady deterioration to apparent stability for months or years, though often ending in a steep decline. Overall, CFA has a median survival of only 3 years. Death commonly results from respiratory failure and/or infection, and there is an increased risk of lung cancer (> 10% of patients). It is not known whether early treatment alters the eventual outcome.

Symptoms and lung function (vital capacity and transfer factor) are monitored but do not accurately reflect the pattern of inflammation/fibrosis in the lung. Ground glass shadowing on HRCT, a cellular biopsy and lymphocytosis at BAL all predict a better response to treatment. Diethylene triamine pentacetic acid (DTPA) scanning is being studied and may predict disease progression.

FA associated with connective tissue disease

FA in systemic sclerosis (FASSc) and RA (RA/FA) is histologically identical to CFA. FASSc has a better prognosis than CFA however, even after controlling for age and presenting lung function. Some studies suggest 20–50% of patients spontaneously improve – a feature not seen in CFA. The clinical course of RA/FA appears similar to CFA, though this is less well studied than FASSc. There are no controlled treatment trials of FA in these diseases. Treatment is as for CFA, therefore.

Bronchiolitis obliterans organizing pneumonia (BOOP)

BOOP (alternative term cryptogenic organizing pneumonitis (COP)) is characterized by buds of granulation tissue in the alveoli (Masson bodies) and inflammatory changes in alveolar walls. BOOP may be associated with connective tissue disorders, drugs and infections, but is frequently of unknown cause. It may also occur seasonally, in spring, suggesting that an inhaled agent may be a cause.

Most commonly, patients are systemically unwell with several weeks of breathlessness and cough. Antibiotics have often been given for presumed infection, without response. Inspiratory crackles, a high ESR and restrictive lung function tests are usual; clubbing and eosinophilia are not.

CXR and HRCT show non-specific non-segmental patchy consolidation, which is often bilateral. Transbronchial biopsy or open lung biopsy is diagnostic. A clinical diagnosis is often made, however, with a characteristic presentation and rapid response to steroids. Most patients respond quickly to steroids, with symptoms improving over days and the CXR clearing over 2 or 3 months. Relapse, with recurrent CXR shadowing, is common and further courses of steroids may be required.

Drugs and radiotherapy

Many drugs cause DPLD, including cytotoxics, amiodarone and nitrofurantoin. Radiation pneumonitis is more likely with concurrent cytotoxic therapy and presents with cough and breathlessness within 2 or 3 months of therapy. Steroids are helpful for both drug-induced and radiation-induced lung disease, but only if given early.

Pulmonary haemorrhage

Many conditions can present with widespread CXR shadowing resulting from diffuse alveolar haemorrhage:

- Haematological (e.g. thrombocytopenia, disseminated intravascular coagulation).
- Connective tissue diseases (e.g. SLE).
- Cardiac (e.g. mitral stenosis, pulmonary oedema).

- Systemic vasculitides.
- Drugs/toxins (e.g. penicillamine).
- Goodpasture's syndrome.
- Idiopathic pulmonary haemosiderosis.

Rare DPLDs

1. Pulmonary Langerhans' Cell Histiocytosis (LCH). LCH (also known as eosinophilic granuloma) may occur alone or as part of multisystem involvement (previously termed histiocytosis X). The cause is unknown. Lung histology shows collections of Langerhans' cells and eosinophils in alveolar and bronchial walls. Langerhans' cells, not normally resident in lungs, contain cytoplasmic organelles (X bodies or Birbeck granules) identified by immunocytochemistry (S-100 antigen). LCH usually presents in males aged 20–40 years. Almost all are current smokers. Most (72%) have breathlessness and cough; other presentations include an abnormal CXR in an asymptomatic patient (23%) and pneumothorax (11%).

The CXR has a nodular appearance, which often affects all zones and may progress to honeycombing. Lytic rib lesions and preserved lung volumes are diagnostic clues. HRCT reveals nodules and thin-walled lung cysts with upper lobe predominance. Initial lung function may show restrictive changes but, later, lung volumes are usually normal or increased owing to gas trapping, with airway obstruction. Before HRCT scanning, diagnosis was usually by surgical biopsy. Electron microscopy identification of Langerhans' cells in BAL fluid is strong evidence of LCH.

Patients must stop smoking. Steroids are often helpful and some respond to immunosuppressants or cytotoxics. Symptoms may also resolve or stabilize spontaneously. Median survival is about 13 years.

2. Lymphangioleiomyomatosis (LAM). LAM is rare, occurring only in women in the reproductive years. Proliferating immature smooth muscle cells infiltrate:

- Alveolar walls, leading to focal emphysema and honeycombing, causing breathlessness and pneumothoraces.
- Pulmonary vessels, leading to haemoptysis.
- Pulmonary lymphatics, leading to chylothoraces and chyloptysis.

Patients usually present with breathlessness, but sometimes with pneumothorax. CXR shows a diffuse distribution of thin-walled lung cysts, but can be normal. Lung function tests show irreversible airway obstruction, similar to that in emphysema. Hormonal influences are probably involved in the aetiology and progesterone has been helpful in treatment. A recent study showed no relationship with oral contraceptive use. Oophorectomy is of no obvious benefit.

3. Idiopathic pulmonary haemosiderosis. A rare disease of childhood or young adulthood. Red cell leakage from pulmonary capillaries into alveoli leads to iron deficiency anaemia, haemoptysis and breathlessness.

4. Alveolar proteinosis (AP). AP may be idiopathic or associated with underlying conditions such as dust exposure (e.g. silica), or haematological malignancy. An intra-alveolar collection of protein and lipid-rich material causes breathlessness, cough and perihilar diffuse CXR shadowing similar to pulmonary oedema.

Diagnosis is by BAL, which produces milky fluid containing eosinophilic material and macrophages. Treatment is by bronchopulmonary lavage to remove the intra alveolar material.

5. Other diseases. Pulmonary infiltrations occasionally occur in a wide variety of other syndromes, including amyloidosis, lipid storage disease, tuberose sclerosis and neurofibromatosis.

Further reading

DuBois RM. Diffuse lung disease: an approach to management. *BMJ*, 1994; **309:** 175–179.
Editorial. Organising pneumonia. COP/BOOP and SOP. *Lancet*, 1992; **340:** 699–700.

Related topics of interest

Imaging techniques (p. 87)
Pulmonary eosinophilia (p. 137)
Pulmonary hypertension (p. 139)
Vasculitis (p. 163)

DIGESTIVE TRACT DISORDERS

Respiratory complications of digestive tract diseases may reflect the proximity of the two systems, for example in oesophageal or hepatic disorders, or multi-system involvment by a systemic process. The symptoms, signs, investigation and management of the respiratory problems are dealt with in the relevant chapters.

Oesophageal disorders

Oesophageal reflux is a common cause of cough. Achalasia of the oesophagus leads to aspiration pneumonia. Systemic sclerosis is associated with FA. Oesophageal rupture is one cause of a pleural effusion or empyema. Carcinoma of the bronchus may compress the oesophagus and cause dysphagia, and distinguishing between a primary oesophageal or lung origin for a malignancy can sometimes be difficult.

Intestinal disorders

Inflammatory bowel disease is associated with pulmonary complications in around 1% of cases. Clubbing is a rare feature of active Crohn's disease. Granulomata are seen in both lung and bowel when Crohn's disease affects the respiratory tract, or if sarcoidosis or tuberculosis involves both organs. Pulmonary hypertension, apical fibrosis, FA, suppurative bronchitis and bronchiectasis are all rare associations of inflammatory bowel disease. Curiously, they may first develop after resection of the affected bowel. Asymptomatic lung function test abnormalities (particularly a low TLCO) are seen in around 10% of patients with inflammatory bowel disease.

Coeliac disease is also associated with FA and haemosiderosis. Any bowel disease that leads to severe hypoproteinaemia may cause pulmonary oedema or pleural effusions. Mesalazine, sulphasalazine and azathioprine can cause pulmonary toxicity.

Pancreatic disorders

Acute pancreatitis results in ARDS in 20% of cases. Chronic pancreatitis is a cause of pleural effusion, an exudate with high amylase. Carcinoma of the pancreas commonly metastasizes to the lungs, either via the blood stream or spread of tumour cells through the diaphragm to cause a pleural effusion. Pulmonary emboli are also common in this disease.

Hepatic disorders

The proximity of the liver to the right lung explains the frequency with which liver disease is associated with problems in the right hemithorax. In addition, several systemic diseases can affect both organ systems.

Clubbing is a rare feature of cirrhosis. Pleural effusion occurs in 5% of patients with cirrhosis, usually in association with ascites. Empyema may be secondary to hepatic or subphrenic abscess. Malignancy commonly spreads from the lungs to the liver and vice versa. The carcinoid syndrome is caused by hepatic metastases from a gut carcinoid tumour. Fibrosing alveolitis is seen in chronic active hepatitis.

Tuberculosis, sarcoidosis and primary biliary cirrhosis all cause pulmonary and hepatic granulomatous lesions. Bronchiolitis is also seen in the Sjogren's-type variant of primary biliary cirrhosis. Suppurative bronchitis and bronchiectasis can complicate sclerosing cholangitis. Cystic fibrosis and alpha-1-antitrypsin deficiency (emphysema, bronchiectasis) affect both lung and liver.

Arterio-venous shunts in the lower lobes cause the 'hepato-pulmonary syndrome' with hypoxaemia which is worse in the upright posture when the increase in perfusion to the lower lobes exaggerates the shunting effect. This is thus one of only a short list of causes of orthodeoxia and platypnoea, with the patient being less breathless when lying down. Pulmonary hypertension is seen in about 1% of patients with cirrhosis and portal hypertension. Failure of the liver to filter vaso-active substances produced in the gastro-intestinal tract has been proposed as a possible mechanism.

Peritoneal disorders   Tuberculosis may affect the peritoneum. Pleural mesotheliomas may extend to the peritoneal cavity, and vice versa.

Further reading

Wagner PD. Impairment of gas exchange in liver cirrhosis. *European Respiratory Journal*, 1995; **8:** 193–195.

Pulmonary complications of systemic disease. In: Murray JF, ed. *Lung Biology in Health and Disease*, vol 59. Marcel Dekker, New York, 1992.

Related topics of interest

DRUG-INDUCED LUNG DISEASE

Many drugs can cause pulmonary disease. Some of the more frequently seen pulmonary diseases caused by drugs are:

- ACE inhibitors: hypersensitivity pneumonitis, interstitial pneumonitis.
- Amiodarone: chronic interstitial pneumonitis, organizing pneumonia.
- Busulphan: pulmonary fibrosis, ARDS.
- Chlorpromazine: drug-induced lupus.
- Diltiazem: drug-induced lupus.
- Gold: interstitial pneumonitis.
- Hydralazine: drug-induced lupus.
- Isoniazid: drug-induced lupus.
- Methotrexate: acute interstitial pneumonitis, asthma, pulmonary fibrosis, pleural effusion.
- Methyl dopa: drug-induced lupus.
- Nitrofurantoin: Type 1 or Type 3 hypersensitivity reactions, chronic hypersensitivity pneumonitis, pleural effusion.
- Paclitaxel: hypersensitivity owing to histamine release, drug-induced pneumonitis.
- Chlorambucil: chronic interstitial pneumonitis.
- Procaineamide: drug-induced lupus.

It should however be noted that this section deals with the idiosyncratic reactions to drugs rather than simple pharmacological effects (e.g. bronchoconstriction caused by β blockers which might be predicted from the pharmacology of the agents). Brief notes are given below on some of the more important drug-induced pulmonary conditions.

Amiodarone

The anti-arythmic amiodarone is an iodinated benzofuran derivative. Pulmonary toxicity occurs in up to 5% of patients and broadly correlates with total cumulative dose, rather than with drug levels measured at an individual time point. The commonest manifestation of amiodarone pulmonary toxicity is chronic interstitial pneumonitis, although organizing pneumonia and ARDS have also been reported.

Typical symptoms of amiodarone-induced chronic interstitial pneumonitis include the insidious onset of breathlessness and a dry cough. The CXR shows diffuse interstitial shadowing. Organizing pneumonia (with or without BOOP) may also occur in a minority of patients with chronic interstitial pneumonitis.

Risk factors for the development of amiodarone-induced pulmonary disease include high doses (>400 mg/day), increasing patient age, long duration of therapy and pre-existing lung disease. However, the condition can occur with lower doses after even short exposure. There are no useful predictors of pulmonary toxicity and practice varies regarding screening for patients taking amiodarone, with some respiratory physicians advocating regular CXRs and/or measurement of transfer factor but others only investigating individuals with increasing breathlessness.

The diagnosis is one of exclusion although the presence of foamy macrophages and a CD8-positive lymphocytosis in lavage fluid is suggestive. Treatment consists of withdrawal of the drug and high-dose steroids for severe cases. Most patients improve if the condition is recognized early.

Chemotherapy and pulmonary toxicity

Many cytotoxic drugs can cause pulmonary toxicity. These include chlorambucil which causes chronic interstitial pneumonitis (<1% of patients) with features similar to the pneumonitis seen with amiodarone. Busulphan causes pulmonary toxicity in approximately 5% of patients, ultimately progressing to pulmonary fibrosis. Pulmonary toxicity has also been reported with many alkylating agents, although it is difficult to know whether these incidences are due to the drug or to underlying disease. Paclitaxel, a recently introduced anti-neoplastic agent derived from the yew, has been reported to cause pulmonary toxicity through two mechanisms: firstly a hypersensitivity reaction possibly resulting from histamine release, and secondly drug-induced pneumonitis.

Methotrexate

The most frequent pulmonary toxicity seen with methotrexate is an acute interstitial pneumonitis although asthma and pulmonary fibrosis have also been reported. Approximately 1–5% of patients are likely to develop methotrexate-induced pulmonary toxicity. There is some evidence that patients with preceding lung disease may be at greater risk of methotrexate-induced pulmonary toxicity. However, with low-dose methotrexate therapy (e.g. in RA) pulmonary toxicity is rare. The clinical and pathological features of methotrexate-induced interstitial pneumonitis are the same as those seen with other causes. Generally patients respond well to withdrawal of methotrexate: high-dose steroids can be used in severe cases, although there are no controlled studies.

Gold

This drug may also cause interstitial pneumonitis.

Nitrofurantoin

The antibiotic nitrofurantoin causes pulmonary toxicity owing to Type 1 or Type 3 hypersensitivity reactions. These are more common in women. Acute hypersensitivity to nitrofurantoin presents with fever, breathlessness, a dry cough and sometimes a rash, usually appearing about 1 week after initial exposure to the drug. Chronic reactions take 1–6 months to develop and present with breathlessness and dry cough but without fever. Common radiological abnormalities include diffuse parenchymal shadowing (predominantly lower zone), occasionally with pleural effusion in patients with acute disease. Patients with chronic disease have more nodular pulmonary shadowing.

Treatment consists of discontinuation of nitrofurantoin and prognosis is good as long as the drug is stopped early, although some patients with more chronic disease may have persistent pulmonary fibrotic change.

ACE inhibitors

ACE inhibitors induce cough in approximately 10% of patients. The cough is dry and often nocturnal. Symptoms regress with cessation of treatment. In addition, these drugs can rarely cause hypersensitivity pneumonitis and interstitial pneumonitis.

Drug-induced lupus

Drug-induced lupus is a syndrome with features similar to SLE. Antihistone antibodies are present in 95% of cases. A large range of drugs have been implicated in drug-induced lupus: the most important are methyl dopa, chlorpromazine, isoniazid, penicillamine, diltiazem, hydralazine, practolol and procaineamide. The majority of patients show similar symptoms to SLE including fever, arthralgia, polyarthropathy, myalgia and rash, but generally without severe multisystem involvement (e.g. renal or CNS disease). The condition usually resolves on cessation of therapy.

Non steroidal anti-inflammatory drugs (NSAIDs) and asthma

Aspirin and other NSAIDs cause acute bronchospasm in a small percentage of asthmatic subjects.

Further reading

Foucher P, Biour M, Blayac JP *et al*. Drugs that may injure the respiratory system. *European Respiratory Journal*, 1997; **10**: 265–279.

Related topics of interest

EMPHYSEMA

Emphysema is a condition in which there is destruction of alveoli. The disease results from chronic inflammatory insults to the lung. Development of emphysema depends upon the interaction of genetic and environmental effects.

Aetiology

1. Alpha-1 antitrypsin deficiency. Alpha-1 antitrypsin is one of the main antiprotease enzymes present in the lung, protecting against degradation of elastin by neutrophil elastase. It is believed that the balance between protease and anti-protease activity is important in preventing lung damage in the context of infection. Hence, individuals with a deficiency of alpha-1 antitrypsin are susceptible to lung damage. The gene for alpha-1 antitrypsin deficiency is situated on chromosome 13. There are a large number of known mutations in the alpha-1 antitrypsin gene, some of which are known to give rise to panacinar emphysema. Individuals who are homozygous for alpha-1 antitrypsin alleles which give rise to normal levels of alpha-1 antitrypsin have the phenotype MM. The commonest deficient allele is the Z allele (2% of the Caucasian population): individuals homozygous for this allele (i.e. ZZ) are at high risk of developing emphysema. The phenotype of these individuals is sometimes called PiZZ (protease inhibitor Z allele). Many other alleles are known, some of which are associated with severe emphysema. Alpha-1 antitrypsin levels can be measured directly in serum: individuals with alpha-1 antitrypsin deficiency will have less than 20% of normal levels, although this does not apply to some of the rarer mutations. Alpha-1 antitrypsin deficiency can present with either respiratory disease or hepatic disease (cirrhosis): the penetration of the respiratory disease is variable but there is marked interaction with cigarette smoking such that individuals with the ZZ genotype who smoke will usually present with severe emphysema in the fourth or fifth decade.

2. Cigarette smoking. Alpha-1 antitrypsin deficiency accounts for 1–2% of patients with emphysema. There is no clear genetic marker for other cases of emphysema, although it is likely that candidate genes (e.g. other anti-protease genes) will become apparent in the near future. Cigarette smoking is therefore the major risk factor for developing emphysema in the population at large.

3. Coal dust. Exposure to coal dust is a recognized cause of emphysema. In practice, most patients (though not all) with emphysema relating to coal dust exposure will also have some evidence of underlying pneumoconiosis. The true contribution of coal dust exposure may be very difficult to ascertain, given that many miners have also smoked.

4. Cadmium. Cadmium exposure is also a risk factor for the development of emphysema.

Pathologically the key feature of emphysema is destruction of alveoli leading to enlarged air spaces within the lung parenchyma and ultimately to hyperinflation. Emphysema frequently co-exists with bullous disease. Two pathological patterns can be identified: panacinar emphysema (associated with alpha-1 antitrypsin deficiency) and centrilobular emphysema.

Clinical features

Typical symptoms include exertional breathlessness, dry cough and wheeze. Breathlessness may not be apparent until there is marked destruction of lung tissue. On examination patients with significant emphysema have hyperinflated lungs with reduced chest expansion (owing to hyperinflation), an increased percussion note, reduced air entry and wheeze.

Investigations

Lung function tests characteristically show airflow obstruction, a reduced transfer factor (owing to alveolar destruction) but increased lung volumes (increased RV and FRC) owing to air trapping. The CXR shows hyperinflation with flattened diaphragms, apparent reduction in cardiac size (in patients without cardiac disease), and hyperlucent lung fields. Many patients have evidence of bullous lung disease. HRCT provides an excellent non-invasive means of diagnosis where there is doubt or where surgery is being considered.

Alpha-1 antitrypsin levels: the normal range is between 1 and 2 units/ml. Patients with alpha-1 antitrypsin deficiency will have levels below the normal range. Because alpha-1 antitrypsin is an acute phase, protein levels rise in the context of infection: measurements should therefore be made when patients are clinically stable.

Management

The most important aspect of management is to stop patients smoking. Drug treatment is the same as for COPD. However, most patients have relatively limited benefit from bronchodilators and/or steroids. Lung reduction surgery may improve both symptoms and lung function in patients with emphysema (see 'chronic obstructive pulmonary disease'). The principle of the operation is to improve the lung mechanics by removing hyperinflated lung. The area of lung to be removed can be defined by the worst affected region on CT scan. Long-term studies are underway to determine if there is a survival benefit from lung reduction surgery. Bullectomy is effective in improving symptoms in patients with large single bullae compressing surrounding lung tissue.

Alpha-1 antitrypsin replacement using aerosolized alpha-1 antitrypsin (derived e.g. from transgenic animals) may prove effective in patients with alpha-1 antitrypsin deficiency, particularly in the context of acute infection. Trials are currently underway utilizing this approach. An alternative replacement approach is to use gene therapy. Pulmonary rehabilitation produces short-term benefits (see 'chronic obstructive pulmonary disease).

Further reading

Mahadeva R, Lomas DA. Alpha-1 antitrypsin deficiency, cirrhosis and emphysema. *Thorax*, 1998; **53:** 501–505.

Related topics of interest

Asthma (p. 17)
Chronic obstructive pulmonary disease (p. 37)

EMPYEMA

Empyema means pus in the pleural space. The most common situation in which an empyema is seen is as a complication of pneumonia. Abscesses in the lung or below the diaphragm can erode into the pleural cavity, but primary infection of the pleural space also occurs.

Aetiology

Pneumonia can be associated with pleural fluid which, in some cases, becomes infected, particularly with *Strep. pneumoniae* or *Klebsiella pneumoniae*. A lung, hepatic or sub-phrenic abscess can rupture into the pleural space to cause an empyema. Primary empyema is usually caused by *Strep. milleri*, but a polymicrobial aetiology with other anaerobic organisms is common. Tuberculosis can infect the pleural space.

Infection may develop after instrumentation of the chest, for example insertion of a chest drain. Post-operatively, an empyema may develop in a pneumonectomy space. Rarer causes are oesophageal rupture, bronchial carcinoma, mesothelioma and actinomycosis. Unusual infections may be seen in the immunocompromized (*Listeria monocytogenes*, *Nocardia asteroides*).

Clinical features

The patient with an empyema is usually unwell and may have rigors and sweating. Pain is common on the affected side. Fever is common. Examination reveals the signs of a pleural effusion (reduced expansion, dull percussion note, diminished tactile vocal fremitus and reduced breath sounds).

Investigations

The CXR shows a pleural effusion; the presence of an air–fluid level suggests an anaerobic organism, a broncho-pleural fistula or an iatrogenic aetiology. Ultrasound scanning can be used to discriminate pleural fluid from inflammatory thickening. In a right-sided empyema an ultrasound scan of the abdomen should be performed if liver function tests are abnormal or if there is any other reason to suspect a sub-phrenic or hepatic abscess.

Blood should be cultured and sent for full blood count, urea, electrolytes, and liver function tests. Pleural fluid should be aspirated for microscopy and culture. Pneumococcal antigen may be present in blood, pleural fluid, saliva or urine. Bronchoscopy should be undertaken if there is suspicion of a proximal bronchial occlusion.

Treatment

Drainage through a large bore intercostal tube is the traditional treatment of an empyema, but smaller bore (12F) 'pig-tail' catheters are equally effective if the fluid is not too viscous. All empyema drains should be put on suction. Smaller bore drains should be flushed with saline every 6 h. Streptokinase appears to speed resolution with minimal risk of bleeding, and should be started immediately after insertion of the drain; each day 250 000 IU are instilled in 20 ml of saline and the tube clamped for 2 h. The drain may be removed when daily drainage is less than 100 ml.

Antibiotic therapy will be guided by culture results but, until these are avaible, a cephalosporin such as Cefuroxime 1.5 g tds IV should be given. Surgical decortication is reserved for chronic loculated collections or if the patient remains unwell despite medical therapy.

Further reading

Davies RJO, Traill ZC, Gleeson FV. Randomised trial of intrapleural streptokinase in community acquired pleural infection. *Thorax*, 1997; **52:** 416–421.

Related topics of interest

ENDOCRINE DISORDERS

Endocrine disease is only rarely associated with respiratory problems, although endocrine abnormalities may be caused by respiratory disease (particularly lung cancer).

Diabetes	Diabetes mellitus is associated with an increased incidence of respiratory infections, including tuberculosis. In ketoacidosis, the characteristic air hunger of Kussmall's respiration is seen in response to the acidosis.
Pituitary	Acromegaly is a cause of OSA, whilst Cushing's disease may be associated with opportunistic lung infection.
Thyroid	Thyrotoxicosis is associated with worsening asthma, and respiratory muscle weakness. Hypothyroidism is associated with improving asthma, respiratory muscle weakness, obstructive and central sleep apnoea and pleural effusion. A goitre may cause upper airway obstruction.
Adrenal	Tuberculosis and lung cancer are causes of Addison's disease. An Addisonian crisis may be precipitated in patients with tuberculosis and borderline adrenal function when they are started on treatment, as a result of liver enzyme induction which increases the metabolism of cortisol. Small-cell lung cancer (SCLC) may secrete adrenocorticotrophic hormone (ACTH) and cause Cushing's syndrome. Adrenal tumours causing Cushing's syndrome may be associated with opportunistic lung infections.

Further reading

Pulmonary complications of systemic disease. In: Murray JF, ed. *Lung Biology in Health and Disease*, vol 59. Marcel Dekker, New York, 1992.

Related topics of interest

EXTRINSIC ALLERGIC ALVEOLITIS

Extrinsic allergic alveolitis (EAA, also known as hypersensitivity pneumonitis) is a reaction characterized by granulomatous inflammation in response to a wide range of agents, predominantly organic dusts, such as spores of fungi and animal proteins. Over 25 causes of EAA have been described. Bird fancier's lung is probably the commonest type, and is usually due to pigeons or budgerigars, though a wide variety of other birds may be responsible, for example parrots or cockatiels. The antigens are the avian serum proteins present on the bloom of birds' feathers and in their excreta. Farmer's lung is due to thermophilic actinomycetes which grow in the heat produced by moulding in damp crops.

Aetiology

Cause	Source	Disease
Bacteria		
Micropolyspora faeni	Mouldy hay	Farmer's lung
Thermoactinomyces vulgaris		
Fungi		
Aspergillus	Mouldy hay	Farmer's lung
Amoebae		
Naegleria gruberi	Contaminated water	Humidifier lung
Animal protein		
Avian protein	Bloom on bird feathers/bird excreta	Pigeon fancier's lung/Budgerigar fancier's lung
Chemical		
Toluene diisocyanate	Paints	EAA due to isocyanates

Pathology and pathogenesis

The presence of serum precipitins (specific IgG) and the time course of acute reactions led to the concept of an immune complex of inhaled antigen and circulating antibody causing alveolitis. The formation of granulomata, however, suggests a cell-mediated T-cell response, not a mechanism mediated by immune complexes. It is now considered that the serum precipitins are merely markers of the disease and are not involved in pathogenesis.

Animal models suggest that in the first 48 h after antigen exposure there is a neutrophil influx, followed by a lymphocyte-predominant alveolitis (often 60% of cells or more). Bronchoalveolar lavage reveals a predominance of CD8 suppressor cells.

The pathology is not pathognomonic and varies with the stage of illness. In acute EAA there is a mononuclear infiltrate of the alveolar walls usually in a bronchocentric distribution, with granulomata (in about 70%) within the inflammation. In subacute or chronic disease (see below for definition) the granulomata are often poorly formed, with inflammation in small airways (respiratory bronchiolitis) and foamy histiocytes in the alveoli. In late disease there is interstitial fibrosis (honeycombing), often without granulomata.

Clinical features

There are two broad types of presentation, acute (usually reversible) and chronic (often poorly reversible). Some authors also describe a sub-acute presentation, but all these forms overlap. Furthermore, a progression from acute to chronic disease with further exposure is certainly not inevitable. In acute EAA, cough and breathlessness together with systemic symptoms (fever, shivers, myalgia) occur 4–12 h after exposure to the antigen. Examination reveals inspiratory crackles and sometimes squeaks, but not wheeze. This type of disease is thought usually to follow acute exposure to a high concentration of antigen (such as in farmer's or pigeon fancier's lung). Without continuing exposure, symptoms settle within a few days. Chronic EAA presents with exertional breathlessness owing to pulmonary fibrosis. There may or may not be a history of previous acute episodes. This type of disease may be due to prolonged low level exposure to antigen – as in budgerigar fancier's lung, for example, which most commonly presents in this form. In acute EAA, examination reveals inspiratory crackles and sometimes squeaks, but not wheeze. In chronic disease, inspiratory crackles are the main sign. Clubbing is rare.

Investigations

In acute EAA the CXR shows small (1–3 mm) nodules commonest in the lowest zones, or diffuse infiltrates, but may be normal. In chronic disease upper- and mid-zone fibrotic disease is characteristic. HRCT is more frequently abnormal than CXR, showing patchy ground-glass shadowing and ill-defined nodules in acute disease in 50–75% of patients. Recently, air trapping has been shown on expiratory HRCT films and is thought to represent disease in small airways. In chronic EAA, HRCT shows fibrosis and irregular opacities but, in contrast to the CXR, shows either mid-zone predominance or no zonal predominance, with some disease occurring in lower lobes similar to CFA.

Both acute and chronic EAA cause restrictive lung function with reduced lung volumes and gas transfer. TLCO is the most sensitive test for monitoring the disease. Acute EAA is accompanied by peripheral blood neutrophilia (not eosinophilia). Appropriate precipitins are found in about 90%, but are also found in over 10% of asymptomatic farmers and 50% of asymptomatic pigeon breeders.

A diagnosis of EAA can be made if there is evidence of exposure to antigen (either on history or as indicated by the presence of precipitins) and compatible symptoms, lung function and radiology. If a diagnosis is not established by these criteria, support is obtained by lymphocytosis on BAL. However, this is not routinely available and more commonly lung biopsy is performed. Transbronchial biopsy is peformed initially but, if unhelpful, thoracoscopic lung biopsy will provide supportive pathology. There is no routine role for inhalation challenge in diagnosis.

Management

Treatment is directed not only to the relief of symptoms in acute episodes but to prevention of long-term pulmonary fibrosis with its associated disability and mortality.

1. Avoidance of antigen. This is superficially attractive, but often problematic. There may be unacceptable consequences from antigen avoidance on livelihood (e.g. for a farmer), or on commitment to a hobby (e.g. pigeon breeders). Furthermore, continued exposure may not lead to further disease in some patients – in one study only one-third of pigeon breeders with continued regular exposure over 10 years had respiratory symptoms. Respiratory protection masks reduce symptoms in pigeon breeders, and those with symptoms should minimize their time in the pigeon loft and reduce high-exposure activities such as cleaning the loft. Likewise better ventilation and more efficient drying of hay before storage reduces the prevalence of farmer's lung. Most farmers will be able to continue their work, particularly if they take measures to reduce exposure.

2. Steroids. There are no controlled trials of therapy. In the acute attack, treatment is unnecessary when recovery is likely with removal from antigen, and the patient is only mildly affected. With progressive disease an initial 1-month trial of high dose prednisolone (40–60 mg) is recommended with gradual reduction over 3–6 months if there is benefit but a more rapid reduction if there is no effect. In acute disease steroids lead to earlier improvement in lung function but do not appear to affect long-term outcome.

Outcome

The risk of developing progressive fibrosis is low, but it is not possible to predict which patients will progress. In the occupational setting, such as farmers with EAA, a reasonable stategy is to monitor lung function at least annually in an attempt to pick up those with progressive functional decline.

Further reading

Hendrick DJ. Extrinsic allergic alveolitis. *Medicine*, 1995; **23:** 352–355.
Bourke S, Boyd G. Pigeon fanciers' lung. *British Medical Journal*, 1997; **315:** 70–71.

Related topic of interest

Diffuse parenchymal lung disease (p. 59)

FIBRE-OPTIC BRONCHOSCOPY

Fibre-optic bronchoscopy is usually performed with the combination of local anaesthesia and light sedation. The scope is passed via the nose or mouth, through the vocal cords and into the trachea. Bronchi can be inspected to the segmental level. Monitoring of oxygen saturation throughout the procedure is recommended. ECG monitoring can be used, but many centres rely on the pulse oximeter to monitor the heart rate. Rigid bronchoscopy is considered under the topic 'Thoracic surgical procedures'.

Fitness for bronchoscopy

The patient's FEV_1 should be at least 0.75 l.

Blood gases are not measured routinely prior to bronchoscopy, unless there are clinical grounds to suspect hypoxia; since bronchoscopy causes a transient fall in PaO_2 of 1–2 kPa, the level before the procedure should be at least 8 kPa (with supplementary oxygen if necessary).

The mortality of bronchoscopy is very low at around 0.01% but, of these deaths, a high proportion are related to cardiac events. Therefore, the test should not be performed within 1 month of a myocardial infarction, or in patients with unstable angina.

Indications

- Slow resolution of pneumonic changes on CXR, to exclude an endobronchial carcinoma.
- Haemoptysis, to identify a source of bleeding.
- Other symptoms such as cough or stridor which could be caused by an endobronchial lesion.
- A central mass on the CXR.
- A peripheral lesion, which is not readily amenable to percutaneous biopsy.
- To remove a plug of mucus or sputum from a patient with a collapsed lobe.
- In anaesthetic practice to facilitate endo-tracheal intubation.
- To obtain specimens for microbiological examination in patients suspected of having TB who do not have sputum, or in immunocompromized patients with CXR changes failing to respond to empirical treatment.

Transbronchial biopsy

Although a fibre-optic scope cannot be passed beyond the level of the sub-segmental bronchus, small forceps can be passed through the scope to more peripheral areas. This is sometimes done under screening to biopsy a mass, but is more commonly employed in the investigation of diffuse lung disease.

Pneumothorax occurs in 5%, requiring intercostal drainage in 1%. Haemorrhage is unusual, but accounts for most of the increase in mortality over simple bronchoscopy to 0.5%. The patient's platelet count and coagulation should be normal.

Small samples of peripheral bronchi and surrounding alveoli are obtained. The technique is best suited to 'bronchocentric' diseases with histological appearances which can be diagnostic on small samples:

- Sarcoidosis.
- Malignancy.
- BOOP.

Bronchoalveolar lavage   Saline is instilled through the bronchoscope whilst it is wedged in a bronchus, to obtain samples from the periphery of the lung. In diffuse lung disease, 150–200 ml are used for differential cell counts and 50–100 ml for infection or suspected malignancy. This is a valuable method of diagnosis in respiratory infections, for example TB, and in the immunocompromized host. Cytology of BAL material can be used to diagnose malignancy, for example bronchoalveolar cell carcinoma or leukaemic pulmonary infiltration. In inflammatory conditions, differential cell counts give an indication of the underlying disease process, but are seldom diagnostic and are not used routinely. Therapeutic BAL is used in alveolar proteinosis.

Further reading

Stradling P. *Diagnostic bronchoscopy*. Churchill Livingstone, Edinburgh, 1991.

Related topics of interest

Biopsy techniques (p. 22)
Lung cancer (p. 97)
Thoracic surgical procedures (p. 154)

HAEMATOLOGICAL DISORDERS

Haematological disorders can affect the lungs in a number of ways:

- Sickle cell anaemia: sickling crises.
- Leukaemia: opportunistic infection, pulmonary haemorrhage, drug-induced lung disease.
- Lymphoma: as for 'leukaemia' plus direct involvement.
- Bleeding diatheses: pulmonary haemorrhage.
- Thrombophilia: thromboembolic disease.
- Myeloma: as for 'leukaemia' plus bone lesions.
- Abnormal white cell function: pulmonary infection, bronchiectasis, pulmonary eosinophilia, plasmacytoma.
- Bone marrow transplant: graft versus host disease.

Many of these areas are dealt with elsewhere in this book. Areas not already covered are dealt with below.

Bone marrow transplantation

Allogeneic bone marrow transplantation is used in acute leukaemia, aplastic anaemia, severe combined immunodeficiency and some chronic leukaemias. Pulmonary complications are the major cause of morbidity and mortality following bone marrow transplantation. The major complications are discussed below.

1. Opportunistic infection. Opportunistic infection is the most frequent post-transplant complication: many organisms cause problems in these patients but overall the most important are probably *Aspergillus* (invasive aspergillosis) and *Pneumocystis carinii*. Patients who are sero-negative for cytomegalovirus (CMV) are also at risk of CMV pneumonitis.

2. Bronchiolitis obliterans. This is much rarer following bone marrow transplantation than following lung transplantation but can occur in relation to chronic graft versus host disease and also following treatment for CMV pneumonitis.

3. Pulmonary oedema. Non-cardiogenic pulmonary oedema has been reported post-bone marrow transplant: the aetiology is unknown.

4. Pulmonary alveolar proteinosis. This disease has been reported rarely following bone marrow transplant.

Sickle cell anaemia and sickling crises

There are a number of sickling disorders, all of which can potentially affect the lungs. The classic sickle cell anaemia (haemoglobin SS) is associated with sickling crises (see below). Sickle cell trait (AS) does not usually produce sickling except in extreme hypoxia. Three other variants are seen: sickle cell haemoglobin C disease (SC) which may produce thrombotic episodes and hence predispose to pulmonary emboli, sickle cell haemoglobin D disease (SD) with similar manifestations to sickle cell anaemia and sickle cell β-thalassaemia (Sβthal) which has a variable clinical spectrum which, at its most severe, resembles sickle cell disease itself.

A sickle crisis is due to acute thrombotic episodes and is usually precipitated by hypoxia or infection. Sickling in the lung presents with acute dyspnoea and often severe pleuritic chest pain causing pulmonary infarction. Patients may be hypoxic, anaemic and have signs of pulmonary infarction. Management consists of admission, intravenous fluid replacement, oxygen and analgesia together with antibiotics if the episode is precipitated by infection (mycoplasma in particular has been associated). Transfusion or partial exchange transfusion may be required for patients who become severely anaemic.

Lymphoma

Both Hodgkin's and non-Hodgkin's lymphoma (both T- and B-cell) can affect the lung in a number of ways, most commonly mediastinal lymphadenopathy or large unilateral pleural effusions owing to obstruction to lymphatic drainage. Lymphoma may arise directly from lymphoid tissue within the lung (primary pulmonary lymphoma); this is rare and usually presents with unresolving consolidation on CXR. Finally, as with all haematological malignancies, the complications of treatment for lymphoma often affect the lung (see above).

Further reading

Pulmonary complications of systemic disease. In: Murray JF, ed. *Lung Biology in Health and Disease*, vol 59. Marcel Dekker, New York, 1992.

Related topic of interest

Immunodeficiency (p. 90)

HAEMOPTYSIS

Haemoptysis is common in the community. Not all patients report it to their general practitioner when it occurs, and only half of those that do are referred for further investigation.

Aetiology

Transient minor haemoptysis is usually related to a respiratory tract infection, such as bronchitis or pneumonia, and settles quickly. Haemoptysis persisting for 2 weeks or more is most likely to be due to lung cancer (40%) or bronchiectasis (40%). Repeated episodes over many years suggest the latter diagnosis. In 10% of cases referred to hospital for further investigation, no cause is found.

Other diseases associated with haemoptysis are bronchial adenoma, inhaled foreign body, AVM, heart failure, pulmonary infarction (vasculitis or embolism), generalized bleeding diatheses, and trauma. Rare causes include aspergilloma, severe systemic hypertension, aortic aneurysms, Goodpasture's syndrome, endometriosis, broncholithiasis, amyloidosis, Ehlers–Danlos and Sjogren's syndromes.

Massive haemoptysis (more than 500 ml in 24 h) is usually due to lung cancer, bronchiectasis, an AVM or a generalized bleeding diathesis.

Investigations

CXR, full blood count (FBC), clotting screen, urea, electrolytes and liver function tests will usually be performed as part of the initial screen. Bronchoscopy will be necessary in most cases, particularly in smokers over the age of 40 years. If this and the CXR are both normal, a HRCT scan should be performed. The combination of HRCT and bronchoscopy will diagnose about 90% of patients with haemoptysis.

Bronchial arteriography is reserved for cases of massive haemoptysis when the bleeding is so vigorous that bronchoscopy is unlikely to be successful in identifying the source of the bleeding. Embolization of the bleeding vessel can be performed at the time of arteriography.

Management

Most cases of haemoptysis settle with no treatment. Patients with massive haemoptysis require bed rest and sedation with an opiate to suppress coughing. If the CXR is abnormal, nursing the patient on their side with the abnormal side down will minimize spill over of blood into the normal lung. Bronchoscopy should be performed within a few days to identify the source of the bleeding.

Bronchial arteriography may be needed if the patient continues to expectorate large volumes of blood, with a view to embolization. Thoracotomy and resection may be required if embolization is not possible or is unsuccessful. Radiotherapy is a useful palliative measure for haemoptysis from a bronchial carcinoma.

Further reading

Toghill PJ. *Examining Patients*. London: Edward Arnold, 1995.
Hempotysis: etiology, evaluation and outcome in a tertiary referral hospital. *Chest*, 1997; **112:** 440–444.

Related topics of interest

Breathlessness (p. 25)
Bronchiectasis (p. 28)
Clinical history (p. 46)
Cough (p. 49)
Lung cancer (p. 97)

HYPERVENTILATION

Hyperventilation can be defined as ventilation which exceeds the rate required for CO_2 elimination.

Aetiology

1. A normal physiological response. Hyperventilation occurs as a normal response to exercise. In addition exposure to high altitude induces hyperventilation: this is apparent following acute exposure to altitudes greater than 2500 m on exercise owing to the reduced PO_2 levels in inspired air. With acclimatization, the respiratory centre is reset but hyperventilation persists. Hyperventilation also occurs in pregnancy.

2. Respiratory disease. Hyperventilation occurs in patients with respiratory disease owing to increased vagal efferent input: these pathways provide information about the state of the lung. The hyperventilation associated with respiratory disease is usually manifested as increased minute ventilation predominantly resulting from an increase in respiratory rate rather than from an increase in tidal volume.

3. Acid base disturbance. Acidosis from any cause results in hyperventilation owing to chemoreceptor input to the respiratory centre. In this case, the pattern of ventilation is different with predominantly an increase in tidal volume without a marked increase in respiratory rate.

4. Central nervous system (CNS) disease. CNS disease, for example a stroke or encephalitis, may affect the respiratory centres and stimulate respiration.

5. Drugs. Salicylates, particularly in overdose, and progesterone can cause hyperventilation.

6. Psychogenic. This is defined as hyperventilation in the absence of underlying physical disease to account for the increased drive to breathe. This occurs in individuals with anxiety who also often have evidence of somatasization. It tends to be episodic (cf. other causes of hyperventilation) and is worse during episodes of anxiety.

Clinical features

The clinical features are due to the changes in acid base balance which hyperventilation induces. Because there is a lag in HCO_3^- transfer across the blood/brain barrier, the cerebrospinal fluid alkalosis is greater than that seen in peripheral blood (where the buffering capacity is higher). Alkalosis has the effect of reducing levels of ionized calcium (binding of calcium to protein being pH-dependent) leading to the classic symptoms of acute hyperventilation which are paraesthesia in the extremities, numbness particularly around the mouth and, in more severe cases, tetany and occasionally seizures. There is some evidence that changes in cerebral blood flow owing to acid base disturbance may also contribute.

The signs present in a patient with hyperventilation will be those of the underlying disorder. In psychogenic cases the hyperventilation may be variable and is frequently associated with sighing respiration, atypical chest pain or tightness, dizziness and palpitations.

Management

Treatment of hyperventilation resulting from underlying disease is that of treating the underlying disease itself. Psychogenic hyperventilation may be difficult to treat. The symptoms of acute hyperventilation (paraesthesia, numbness, tetany) can be reversed by rebreathing, classically using a paper bag. The rebreathing of CO_2 leads to a rise in $PaCO_2$ and hence the reversal of the pH changes. Reassurance coupled with an explanation of the cause of the symptoms of hyperventilation syndrome may help. In the longer term, teaching patients how to control their breathing during episodes of anxiety is effective in at least some individuals, together with treatment of any underlying psychiatric condition. This may prove difficult, although agents such as sertraline and the use of cognitive behavioural therapy may be beneficial.

Further reading

Gardner WN. The pathophysiology of hyperventilation disorders. *Chest* 1996; **109:** 516–534.

Related topic of interest

Breathlessness (p. 25)

IMAGING TECHNIQUES

In addition to the CXR, other imaging techniques are often required, either for diagnostic purposes or to give more precise anatomical detail. These are considered in this chapter.

Computerized tomography

Conventional CT scans of the chest usually image slices of the chest which are 1 cm in thickness. They can be confined to areas of interest, or taken contiguously to cover the lung in its entirety. CT is used in the following situations:

- To clarify if a pulmonary or mediastinal lesion is present when the CXR is equivocal, for example when a question has been raised about hilar enlargement.
- To assess the mediastinum in the assessment of operability of proven or suspected lung cancer. The scan will usually be extended caudally to include the liver and adrenals, both common sites of metastases from carcinoma of the bronchus.
- To define the exact anatomy of a mediastinal lesion, prior to biopsy or resection.
- To detect pulmonary metastases which may be invisible on the plain CXR.
- Suspected aortic aneurysm.
- Spiral CT, which can produce a CT pulmonary angiogram with the injection of contrast media to detect pulmonary emboli.
- Pleural disease. Lesions such as plaques which may be difficult to see on a CXR are readily defined on CT. Pleural effusions can be differentiated from pleural thickening, and the presence of loculations easily demonstrated. Infolding of the lung secondary to pleural thickening can mimic an intra-pulmonary mass on a CXR, but on CT appearances of vessels curving round and into the lesion is characteristic. Occasionally, CT may be helpful in the management of a difficult pneumothorax.

High resolution computerized tomography

HRCT involves reconstructing images of thin (1–2 mm) slices of the lungs. These slices are spaced at regular intervals, often 1 cm, throughout the lungs. The following are examples of diseases with characteristic HRCT appearances:

- Bronchiectasis: a dilated bronchus seen in cross-section is larger than its accompanying vessel, giving an appearance known as a signet-ring. When cut longitudinally a tram-line appearance is seen. Bronchiectasis is seen on the CXR in 90% of cases but, if there is a suggestive history but a normal CXR, then HRCT should be performed. It will also define the extent of disease when resection is being considered.

- FA: sub-pleural linear shadows are seen in the lower part of the lungs in early disease. Atelectasis in the most dependant part of the lung can cause similar appearances but, unlike fibrosis, such changes disappear if the patient is scanned in the prone rather than the supine position. Reticular and honeycomb changes are often associated with ground-glass opacification.
- EAA: patchy inflammatory infiltrates or ground glass opacities. If a scan is then taken during expiration, obstruction of bronchioles prevents lobules from emptying and these then appear as dark segments on the scan.
- Sarcoidosis: nodules situated along the broncho-vascular bundles, predominantly in the mid- and upper-zones. Later conglomerate masses occur. Mediastinal lymphadenopathy is common.
- Lymphangitis carcinomatosa: thickening of the interlobular septa and fissures.
- Emphysema and bullae.

Magnetic resonance imaging

At the time of writing, MRI of the lungs is in its infancy. However, it is rapidly becoming apparent that this technique is an excellent method of imaging the pulmonary vasculature and may become the investigation of choice for pulmonary emboli and also for demonstrating the aorta.

Radionuclide scans

Ventilation/perfusion (V/Q) scans utilize different isotopes to assess the ventilation and perfusion of different regions of the lung. Ventilation scanning involves inhalation of a technetium-99m aerosol or the gases xenon-133 or krypton-81m. Perfusion is measured by intravenous injection of technetium-99m macroaggregates or microspheres.

In the assessment of pulmonary emboli, V/Q scans are reported as low, high or intermediate probability. Many other diseases, such as COPD, asthma, pneumonia and FA, alter ventilation and perfusion, making interpretation of the scans difficult.

Gallium-67 scans show areas of active inflammation in sarcoidosis, but add little diagnostic information and are not used routinely. Technetium-99m-labelled particles in the form of an aerosol can be used to assess muco-ciliary clearance.

Pulmonary angiography

Pulmonary angiography involves the passage of a catheter from a large vein through the right heart and into the pulmonary artery. Injection of contrast then outlines the pulmonary arterial tree. It has a mortality of around 0.5%. It is widely regarded as the gold standard for the diagnosis of pulmonary embolism. It is also used to demonstrate AVM, which can also be obliterated using a variety of agents inserted through the catheter into the feeding vessel.

Bronchial arteriography
Patients with severe haemoptysis may need to undergo bronchial arteriography to identify the site of the bleeding, with a view to embolization during the procedure or surgical resection. A catheter is passed retrogradely from the femoral artery into the aorta and thence into the bronchial arteries. These usually arise directly from the aorta, but vary in number and may arise from the intercostal arteries. The bronchial circulation also receives smaller branch vessels from the mediastinum, so identifying the vessel feeding a site of bleeding may be difficult.

Ultrasound
Air does not transmit ultrasound, so thoracic ultrasound is confined to the investigation of the pleural space or lesions immediately underneath the parietal pleura. In patients with CXR evidence of pleural shadowing it will distinguish between thickening and fluid, and detect the presence of loculations within pleural fluid. The optimal site for aspiration can be easily identified.

Ultrasound scanning can also be used to image an elevated diaphragm, to see if it moves normally or if it is paralysed. Paradoxical motion should be defined as upward motion of the hemidiaphragm of at least 2 cm on inspiration.

Further reading

Armstrong P, Wastie ML. *Diagnostic Imaging*. Blackwell, Oxford, 1998.
Bittner RC, Felix R. Magnetic resonance (MR) imaging of the chest: state-of-the-art. *European Respiratory Journal*, 1998; **11:** 1392–1404.

Related topics of interest

Chest X-ray (p. 31)
Fibre-optic bronchoscopy (p. 79)

IMMUNODEFICIENCY

The general approach to immunocompromized patients is considered first and then the specific problems associated with HIV. Immunocompromized states may be congenital or acquired, the latter being much more common. It must be remembered that many other factors apart from the immune system are important in protecting the lung, including mechanical factors (e.g. the epiglottis), the gag and cough reflexes, the mucociliary escalator, macrophages and proteins secreted in the respiratory tract.

Aetiology

Diagnosis of lung disease in these patients is a major challenge. When faced with a breathless patient with CXR shadowing and fever the differential is large, but may be subdivided according to the pathogenesis:

- Infection: (see below).
- Underlying disease process: (e.g. infiltration in leukaemia, lymphoma).
- Treatment: cytotoxics, radiation, white blood cell transfusion.
- Associated consequences of the underlying disease, infection or treatment, including haemorrhage, oedema.

In an immunocompromized patient the potential pathogens are related to the type of immune defect:

- Neutrophil defect (e.g. chronic granulomatous disease, leukaemia, cytotoxic drugs): bacteria (gram positive or negative) and fungi (e.g. *Aspergillus*).
- Immunoglobulin deficiency (e.g. congenital IgA or IgG deficiency, myeloma): bacteria (*Strep. pneumoniae, Haemophilus influenzae*).
- T-cell defect (e.g. congenital thymic aplasia, cytotoxics, AIDS): bacteria, pneumocystis carinii, mycobacteria, viruses (e.g. CMV), parasites.

Clinical features

Most commonly it is known or suspected that the patient is immunocompromized, but recurrent or unusual lung infections must raise the possibility of immunocompromize even when this has not been suspected previously. Clinical pointers to the diagnosis are:

- Clinical setting (e.g. if on cytotoxics: must consider drug-induced disease).
- Time course of the illness (e.g. insidious onset: pneumococcal pneumonia unlikely).
- Time relationship to treatment (e.g. 2 months after organ transplant: consider CMV).
- Status of underlying disease (e.g. in lymphoma, lung

involvement is unlikely if the disease is under control elsewhere).

- Review of fluid charts (excess fluids raise possibility of pulmonary oedema).
- Fever (suggests infection but drugs can also cause).
- Haemoptysis (suggests haemorrhage or infarction though infection can also cause).
- Past history of tuberculosis.
- Pleurisy (unlikely in *Pneumocystis carinii* pneumonia (PCP) or oedema).
- Associated systemic symptoms (e.g. arthralgia with CMV).
- Pointers suggesting HIV (gay, bisexual, IV drug use, sex in high HIV prevalence area, blood transfusion, haemophilia).

Examination is often unhelpful diagnostically. Signs of cardiac failure and systemic disease should be sought.

Investigations

The CXR often shows non-specific diffuse shadowing. Cardiomegaly and septal lines suggest cardiac failure. Acute illness with lobar or segmental shadowing points to bacterial pneumonia. Multifocal shadows are usually seen with fungi. A V/Q scan is necessary if pulmonary embolism is suspected and CT may be characteristic in invasive aspergillosis.

Sputum, urine and blood cultures together with pleural specimens should be obtained for microscopy, culture and detection of specific antigen. If at this stage the clinical impression is that of acute bacterial pneumonia, then broad spectrum antibiotics should be started.

Invasive investigation is frequently necessary when there is (a) diffuse CXR shadowing, (b) likelihood of opportunist infection, (c) lack of response to initial treatment, (d) doubt as to the underlying process.

- BAL is safe and diagnostic in more than 60% of cases with a much higher rate where infection is the cause. Bronchoscopy can be performed with supplemental oxygen if necessary but, if the pace of the illness suggests ventilation is imminently required, it is safer to intubate before bronchoscopy.
- Transbronchial biopsy usually adds little to BAL and carries risks of haemorrhage and pneumothorax. It is useful in the diagnosis of malignancy and drug-induced shadowing.
- Open lung biopsy (OLB) is diagnostic in 60–90% in various series but complications occur in at least 10%, including death. Whether OLB affects outcome in these ill patients is controversial.

- Percutaneous fine needle aspirate is appropriate for focal lesions.

Very close liaison with microbiology laboratories is essential in the handling and interpretation of specimens.

Specific conditions/ organisms

1. Bacterial pneumonia. If the clinical picture suggests pneumonia owing to pathogenic organisms, antibiotics need to cover *Streptococcus pneumoniae, Haemophilus influenzae, Staphylococcus aureus* and gram negative organisms. Cefuroxime and gentamicin is an appropriate regime.

2. Tuberculosis. TB may be of rapid and diffuse onset (in contrast to the immunocompetent patient) and is particularly likely in those with a history of TB or from high-prevalence regions. Standard anti-TB therapy is usually successful.

3. Cytomegalovirus. CMV typically causes diffuse pneumonitis 6–8 weeks after transplantation and may be reactivation or primary infection. Antigenic change in affected cells can be identified in BAL before culture is available. Intravenous ganciclovir is the treatment of choice.

4. Nocardia. This may be associated with skin and brain lesions. Cotrimoxazole is effective.

5. Fungi. PCP is discussed in the section on HIV. In other immunocompromized patients the onset is often more acute and treatment shorter as immunosuppression may be less prolonged. Aspergillus may cause invasive disease. Cryptococcus frequently causes single or multiple nodules, sometimes with effusion. There may be accompanying meningitis. The organism is identified by India ink stain. Mucormycosis is often rapidly fatal and associated with sinus disease in diabetics.

HIV and the lung

The lung is frequently involved. Common infecting organisms at increasing levels of immunosuppression are:

- Bacterial pneumonia (throughout the course of the disease).
- *M. tuberculosis* (mid-course sentinel infection).
- PCP (late – usually CD4 cell count <200).
- *M. avium* intracellulare (late – usually CD4 <50).

Many other opportunistic organisms affect the lung less commonly. Lung involvement is also seen in Kaposi's sarcoma, lymphoma, lymphocytic and non-specific interstitial pneumonitis.

1. Pneumocystis carinii pneumonia. Molecular biology techniques show that *Pneumocystis carinii* is a fungus. The incidence of PCP has declined since prophylaxis has become widespread but it remains the most common opportunist lung infection in HIV in the developed world.

Characteristically, there is gradual onset of cough, breathlessness and malaise over several weeks, with fever, tachypnoea and signs of immunosuppression (e.g. oral candida). Crackles are uncommon. CXR usually shows diffuse bilateral perihilar shadowing. In 10% of cases the CXR is normal and atypical presentations include focal consolidation and cavitation. Pneumothorax occurs in 6%, but pleural effusion or glands suggest alternative or coexistent diagnoses.

Hypoxia is common at presentation. Desaturation on exercise is a sensitive screening test. Where necessary, BAL is the procedure of choice, being diagnostic for PCP in more than 90% of cases. In specialist centres, induced sputum achieves a high diagnostic yield. Transbronchial biopsy (TBB) adds only marginally and in view of additional morbidity is not performed unless other diagnoses are likely. PCR is likely to enhance the sensitivity of BAL. With a typical clinical picture, treatment is often started empirically, and bronchoscopy reserved for patients not responding by 5–7 days.

First line therapy is high-dose cotrimoxazole, initially IV and then oral (or oral throughout in mild cases) for 3 weeks. Drug toxicity is commoner in HIV patients (rash, bone marrow suppression). Second line therapies include oral dapsone and trimethoprim, and IV or nebulized pentamidine. High-dose steroids, for example methyl prednisolone, are of proven value in initial treatment of severe disease.

Mortality from the first episode is around 10%. Opinion has varied as to the appropriateness of mechanical ventilation. In a Paris study, there was a 50% survival with ventilation early in the course of PCP, but a 96% mortality when treatment had already been given for 5–7 days. If support is needed, it is reasonable to consider early ventilation in a first episode of PCP.

2. Other infections. Bacterial pneumonia is commoner in HIV-positive patients and may be recurrent. Tuberculosis is the commonest lung complication in sub-Saharan Africa and Asia. It is due to reactivated disease, reflecting the high prevalence in these areas. Unusual features are common, for example tuberculin negative, lower zone shadows, smear negative disease and extra pulmonary features. Mycobacterium tuberculosis (MTB) may accelerate the course of HIV. There is usually a good response to standard treatment. Isoniazid is then usually given permanently.

Mycobacterium avium intracellulare may occur in more than 50% of cases in late disease, usually with disseminated disease. Unusually for mycobacteria, blood cultures may be positive. Combinations of rifabutin, clarithromycin, ciprofloxacin, clofazamine and ethambutol may control but not cure disease.

CMV is found in BAL in up to 50% of HIV-positive patients but rarely causes pneumonia. If CMV pneumonia is strongly suspected, lung biopsy is needed to look for cytopathological evidence of infection.

3. *Kaposi's sarcoma (KS)*. KS occurs predominantly in homosexual men. CXR shows nodular or perihilar densities, and pleural effusions (in up to 50%). Over 50% have KS lesions elsewhere (e.g. skin, pharnyx). Combination chemotherapy may palliate.

4. *Pneumonitis*. Both lymphocytic (mostly children) and non-specific (adults) interstitia pneumonitis are of unknown aetiology and may respond to steroids.

Prophylaxis

1. *Pneumocycstis carinii*. Primary prophylaxis is commonly used with long-term immunosuppression and, in leukaemia, chemotherapy. In HIV, prophylaxis is started with CD4 counts of greater than 200 or with an AIDS-defining diagnosis irrespective of the CD4 count. Secondary prophylaxis after PCP is always given in AIDS, and in other immunocompromized patients depending on the anticipated subsequent immunosuppression. Oral cotrimoxazole (e.g. two tablets od or bd three times a week) is the most effective prophylaxis. Dapsone and/or pyrimethamine or nebulized pentamidine (in HIV) are less effective.

2. *MTB*. Primary prophylaxis is considered for immunocompromised patients with previous tuberculosis or in those from a high-prevalence area. In the USA isoniazid prophylaxis is recommended in HIV patients with a positive tuberculin test.

3. *CMV.* Vaccination may be given in seronegative potential transplant recipients.

Further reading

Mitchell DM. AIDS and the lung. *Medicine*, 1995; **23**: 318–321.

Related topics of interest

LUNG ABSCESS

A lung abscess is localized infection of the lung with necrosis. Air is seen within the destroyed area if gas-forming bacteria are present, but also if the necrotic tissue ruptures into a bronchus. This gives the characteristic CXR appearance of a thick-walled cavity with an air–fluid level.

Aetiology

Staphylococcus aureus, *Klebsiella pneumoniae* and anaerobic bacteria (*Streptococcus milleri, Bacteroides*) are the main causes of lung abscesses. Mycobacterium tuberculosis should always be considered as a possible cause in any cavitating lesion. The presence of multiple abscesses in the lungs suggests a blood-borne aetiology, such as right-sided endocarditis.

Clinical features

The patient with a lung abscess will feel unwell with general malaise, rigors and sweating. They usually have a cough productive of sputum, which may generate an unpleasant taste in the mouth. Apart from fever, there may be few abnormal physical signs. If the abscess is adjacent to the pleura, there may be dullness to percussion and reduced breath sounds.

Investigations

As with any serious lung infection, blood should be sampled for a full blood count, urea, electrolytes, liver function tests and blood cultures. The CXR appearances mentioned above are characteristic. The differential diagnosis of air within a lung shadow is:

- Cavitating pneumonia (may be multiple cavities).
- Pulmonary infarction (pulmonary embolus).
- Vasculitis (Wegener's granulomatosis).
- Sterile fluid within an area of lung destroyed by pneumonia (pneumatocoele).
- Infection within a pre-existing cavity such as a bulla.
- Aspergilloma.
- Lung cancer, particularly squamous.
- Progressive massive fibrosis.
- Rheumatoid nodule.

If available, sputum should be cultured and, if the cause is not identified, material from within the abscess should be obtained either by bronchoscopy with BAL or percutaneous needle aspiration.

Management

Antibiotics are the mainstay of therapy. If the patient is toxic and unwell, an intravenous cephalosporin such as Cefuroxime 1.5 g tds IV should be given together with Metronidazole 400 mg tds PO. Amoxycillin 500 mg tds or 3 g bd PO, together with Metronidazole 400 mg tds PO, is adequate therapy for most patients. The choice of antibiotics may be influenced by culture and sensitivity results when these become available. Antibiotics should be continued for at least 2 weeks, and longer if the CXR shows incomplete resolution. Percutaneous or surgical drainage of a lung abscess is seldom necessary.

Complications Rupture of the abscess into the pleural space causes an empyema. Metastatic abscess may develop by blood-borne spread.

Further reading

Neild JE, Eykyn SJ, Phillips I. Lung abscess and empyema. *Quarterly Journal of Medicine*, 1985; **57**: 875–882.

Related topics of interest

Empyema (p. 72)
Mycobacteria (p. 105)
Pneumonia (p. 124)

LUNG CANCER

Lung cancer is the commonest malignancy in the Western World. In the UK it was responsible for 41 000 deaths in 1991, about 70% of which were in males. Of all males, 8% die of lung cancer as do 4% of females, with an overall threefold increase since 1950. Mortality rates are beginning to decline in men but continue to increase in women such that in some areas female mortality from the disease has overtaken that from breast cancer.

The WHO classification, and frequency of occurrence from a study in Edinburgh are as follows:

Squamous	48%
Small cell	24%
Adenocarcinoma	13%
Large cell	10%
Other	5%

Aetiology

Tobacco smoking is responsible for about 85% of all types of lung cancer with the exception of adenocarcinoma. Environmental tobacco smoke (passive smoking), certain occupational exposures (e.g. asbestos, nickel), and air pollution (urban environment) are all associated with increased risk of lung cancer, as is FA. Genetic and dietary factors are likely to be important.

Clinical features

Patients present with, or develop, symptoms and signs owing to four main effects of cancer.

1. Those resulting from the primary cancer. Cough is the presenting symptom in over 50% of patients, and haemoptysis or breathlessness in about 25%. Breathlessness is usually due to bronchial obstruction or a pleural effusion. Chest or back pain is due to local invasion of pleura, ribs or spine (secondary deposits in these sites cause similar pain). Pain along the inner arm may be due to brachial plexus involvement from an apical (Pancoast) cancer. Unilateral monophonic wheeze is a sign of partial major airway obstruction.

2. Those resulting from mediastinal invasion or spread. Hoarseness suggests recurrent laryngeal nerve involvement, and dysphagia suggests oesophageal compression by glands. Superior vena caval obstruction (SVCO) causes facial swelling, non-pulsatile neck veins and dilated veins on the upper chest wall. A paralysed diaphragm is likely to be due to phrenic nerve involvement and Horner's syndrome to sympathetic trunk involvement at C_8T_1. Arrhythmias or pericardial effusion can be due to cardiac involvasion.

3. Those resulting from distant spread. Supraclavicular glands are involved in 30%. One-third of patients present with symptoms/signs owing to distant spread, predominantly bone, brain or liver. Bony secondaries can cause pain, or hypercalcaemia with associated constipation, nausea, thirst and confusion.

4. Non-metastatic effects. Systemic symptoms, for example poor appetite and weight loss, occur in more than 50% at presentation. Clubbing is present in about 20% and occasionally associated with hypertrophic pulmonary osteoarthropathy (HPOA), which presents with pains in the wrists and ankles and which may be misdiagnosed as a form of arthritis. Both clubbing and HPOA mainly occur in squamous cancer. A wide variety of neuromyopathies have been described in association with lung cancer, including the Eaton–Lambert syndrome. Hypercalcaemia, occurring in absence of bone secondaries, is due to parathyroid hormone-like peptides, a phenomenon seen in about 6% of squamous cancer. Antidiuretic hormone secretion is a feature of SCLC, occurring in 12% in one series. Clinical effects are those of hyponatraemia. ACTH secretion is also seen in SCLC but clinical effects are relatively rare, probably because the poor prognosis of SCLC does not allow manifestations of Cushing's syndrome to develop.

Investigations

Investigation has two roles: (a) to confirm the diagnosis of lung cancer and the cell type and (b) to stage the disease. Both are important if appropriate treatment and prognosis are to be given, though there will be a small number of patients for whom a clinical/radiographic diagnosis will be appropriate.

1. CXR. The common appearances are of a mass, pleural effusion, bulky hilum, collapse, poor resolution of consolidation and lymphangitis carcinomatosa. A normal CXR does not exclude a central cancer. Appearances do not correlate with the cell type, though a cavitating peripheral mass is usually a squamous cancer.

2. Bronchoscopy. FOB is the investigation of choice for central cancers. Of all lung cancers, 70% will be diagnosed at this investigation. Biopsies for histology and samples for cytology are taken, and an assessment of operability made (how close the cancer is to the main carina, and whether there are sub-carinal glands). Rigid bronchoscopy under general anaesthetic may be necessary for major tracheal cancers or where bleeding is a problem and control of the airway with better suction is a necessity.

3. Percutaneous needle biopsy (PCNB). This is the appropriate investigation for peripheral cancers and is a radiological technique under fluoroscopic or CT control. Opinion varies as to the need for PCNB for a lesion which is likely to be cancer in a patient who is otherwise operable. Provided a cutting needle is used to obtain the histology a significant number of positive benign diagnoses will be made.

4. Sputum cytology. This is used less than other techniques because of its lower sensitivity for diagnosis of lung cancer in general and its poorer accuracy in the identification of cell type. It is valuable however in patients for whom FOB/PCNB are not appropriate.

5. Other biopsies. Biopsy or aspiration at other involved sites (pleura, neck glands, liver) may be helpful.

In addition to these diagnostic tests, patients with lung cancer should have a full blood count, urea, electrolytes liver function tests, and calcium measured. These are important in prognosis, in identifying metastatic spread and in planning treatment. In addition, the three main hormone-related paraneoplastic syndromes can be identified.

Staging

Staging of the disease is vital to define appropriate management. All patients should be considered initially for surgery, though operable SCLC is rare. Two questions need to be asked: firstly, is the patient fit enough for surgery? Points to consider are:

- Lung function. Surgery is not usually possible if the FEV is less than 1.5L for lobectomy or 2.0L for pneumonectomy.
- Cardiac status. Current ischaemic heart disease (severe angina, myocardial infarction within 6 weeks) is a contra-indication.
- Age of itself is not a bar to surgery.
- Other systemic illnesses.
- The patient's wishes.

The second question is whether resection is likely to be curative. Clinical assessment may have already revealed mediastinal or other spread contra-indicating surgery. If not, and the patient is fit enough for surgery, then a CT of thorax and upper abdomen should be performed to assess the mediastinum and the possibility of liver and adrenal metastases. If CT is normal the patient can proceed to thoracotomy. If mediastinal glands are seen, larger than 1–1.5 cm, these need to be sampled at mediastinoscopy, as even large glands may not be malignant but merely reactive. CT brain and bone scanning are not routinely performed unless symptoms or biochemistry suggest metastases.

1. Non-SCLC. The staging system used is based on the TNM classification from Stage 1 (tumour <3 cm in size and distal to lobar bronchus without spread) to Stage 4 (distant spread).

2. SCLC. Staging in SCLC divides patients into two categories:

- Limited disease – cancer confined to the hemithorax and ipsilateral supraclavicular glands (30%).
- Extensive – all other patients.

Treatment

1. Surgery. The aim of surgery is cure. Perioperative mortality resulting from pneumonectomy is 5–8% and for lobectomy 2–3%, increasing in those patients over 70 years of age to 6–10% and 5–7%, respectively, though curative resections can certainly be performed in elderly patients.

2. Radiotherapy (R/T). Radical radiotherapy is given with intent to cure or at least to provide long-term local control. Patients with non-SCLC, inoperable for medical reasons, should be considered for radical R/T. This is only suitable for relatively small cancers (<6 cm in size) encompassable in a radiotherapy field. Palliative radiotherapy (generally one or two fractions) provides good symptom relief in both non-SCLC and SCLC for haemoptysis, SVCO, cough, and bone pain.

3. Chemotherapy. This is the first-line treatment for SCLC. It improves survival and quality of life with an important role in symptom palliation. An example of a currently employed regime for relatively fit patients is adriamycin, cyclophosphamide and etoposide given every 3 weeks for 6 cycles.

The role of chemotherapy in non-SCLC is currently under debate. Several agents show activity in the disease, and a recent meta analysis confirms a survival advantage for cisplatin-based regimes. As yet, data on quality of life are lacking.

Outcome

1. SCLC. Untreated patients with limited disease have a median survival of 12 weeks and those with extensive disease 4 weeks. With chemotherapy median survival improves to around 12–15 months and 6–8 months, respectively, and with modern regimes and antiemetics the quality of life during this period is frequently good.

2. Non-SCLC. Of all patients, 80% are clinically inoperable and a further 10% will be inoperable after mediastinal evaluation with CT and mediastinoscopy. In those undergoing surgery there is a 40% 5-year survival. The overall 5-year survival for all patients with non-SCLC is about 5%. Prognosis strongly relates to stage, with 5-year survival for Stage 1 cases treated surgically being 55–70%, while the median survival for inoperable patients treated is 6–9 months with only a 1% 5-year survival. Radical radiotherapy can achieve 5-year survivals of 20–30% in Stage 1 disease. Fractionation of treatment given several times a day further improves survival.

Further reading

Souhami R. Lung cancer. *British Medical Journal*, 1992; **304:** 1298–1301.
Plant P, Muers MF. Investigation and staging of lung cancer. *British Journal of Hospital Medicine*, 1996; **55:** 627–630.
Morgan WE. The surgical management of lung cancer. *British Journal of Hospital Medicine*, 1996; **55:** 631–634.
Macbeth F. Radiotherapy in the treatment of lung cancer. *British Journal of Hospital Medicine*, 1996; **55:** 639–642.

Related topics of interest

LUNG FUNCTION TESTS

Lung function tests are central to the management of many respiratory conditions. They are used in establishing a diagnosis, assessing severity, and monitoring progression and the response to treatment. This chapter will discuss the more commonly used lung function tests.

The values recorded for most of these tests depend upon the sex of the patient, their age and their height. Predicted values appropriate to the patient population are needed for comparison. To define the normal range for lung function tests, 80% to 120% predicted is often used, although the Standardized Residual (SR) has more scientific validity. This is calculated by subtracting the predicted value from the observed, and dividing the result by the residual standard deviation of the prediction equation. Normal test results have a SR within ±1.64.

Peak expiratory flow rate (PEFR)

Monitoring of PEFR is used in the management of asthma, for diagnosis, assessment of severity and response to treatment. However, it is important to remember that a low PEFR is not diagnostic of airflow obstruction, but is also seen in some restrictive conditions with a low vital capacity when the patient cannot take a deep breath in before blowing into the peak flow meter. The characteristic pattern of a PEFR which varies both within and between days (by more than 15% of the mean PEFR) is nevertheless a useful pointer to the diagnosis of asthma.

Spirometry

Spirometry is measurement of the vital capacity (VC) and the volume expired during the first second of a forced expiration (FEV$_1$). FEV$_1$ is one of the most reproducible lung function tests, more reliable than PEFR in airflow obstruction, and a strong predictor of mortality. In obstructive problems, the FEV$_1$ is low and the ratio of FEV$_1$ to VC is reduced; the VC itself may also be low, but not to the same extent as FEV$_1$. In a restrictive process the FEV$_1$ and VC are both low, with the ratio of FEV$_1$ to VC being normal or even high.

Reversibility

It is common practice in respiratory clinics and lung function laboratories to test for reversibility of airflow obstruction to inhaled bronchodilators, although there is only poor correlation with how the patient will respond symptomatically when using the same medication at home over a longer period. Repeat testing is normally performed 15–20 min after administration of a short-acting beta-agonist, or 30–40 min for an anti-cholinergic. The variability of FEV$_1$ and VC is such that any change after administration of a bronchodilator must be greater than 200 ml and 350 ml, respectively, to be significant. When PEFR is used to test for reversibility, the increase should be at least 60 l/min to be significant.

Bronchial reactivity

In patients suspected of having asthma who have non-diagnostic spirometry and serial peak flow monitoring, the reaction of the airways to increasing concentrations of a bronchoconstrictor agent, such as histamine or methacholine, can be measured. The response is expressed as the concentration or dose required to produce a 20% fall in FEV_1. This should be more than 8 mg/l or 4 μmol, depending upon which test technique is used; values lower than this indicate abnormally reactive airways.

Flow-volume loops

A flow-volume trace is particularly valuable in the diagnosis of upper airway obstruction, although it also shows characteristic abnormalities in a number of other diseases. In a normal subject, the inspiratory part of the loop is convex, whereas the expiratory loop is concave, particularly at lower lung volumes when flow is limited by airway closure. The variation of flow with lung volume is lost when there is an upper airway problem, so flat plateaux are seen on the flow-volume loop. With a rigid lesion in the upper airway, plateaux are seen on both inspiratory and expiratory flow, and the loop assumes a box-like shape. If the lesion is less rigid and above the sternal notch, flow is limited during inspiration, but is more normal during expiration when the positive pressure within the airway causes the narrowed segment to dilate. In contrast, with a lesion below the sternal notch the narrowing is worse during expiration, but alleviated during inspiration when the airway is enlarged by the effect of the negative intra-thoracic pressure which surrounds it. Numerical indices calculated from the trace are less helpful than visual inspection.

Lung volumes

In a restrictive process, TLC, RV and FRC are all low. The cause of the reduction in lung volume may be stiffness of the lungs, stiffness of the chest wall, or weakness of the respiratory muscles.

In obstruction the lung volumes may be normal or high, and the values obtained are also influenced by the technique used to measure them – helium dilution or body plethysmography. The elevation of lung volumes is partly due to loss of lung elastic recoil, and partly to airway collapse which prevents the lung from emptying.

Carbon monoxide transfer factor (TLCO)

Carbon monoxide travels from the alveoli to the capillaries at much the same rate as oxygen. The TLCO measures the rate of diffusion of this gas from the inspired air through the lungs and into the pulmonary circulation, where it combines with haemoglobin. Because there are several phases to this process, several different disease processes can cause a low TLCO: resection of a lung, emphysema, most causes of DPLD (e.g. FA), pulmonary vasculitis, or oligaemia (right to left shunts) and anaemia for example. TLCO should always be corrected for the haemoglobin concentration. A high TLCO is seen in pulmonary haemorrhage, when there is an abundant supply of haemoglobin with which carbon monoxide can combine.

Carbon monoxide transfer coefficient

The KCO is the TLCO divided by the size of the lungs. It usually changes in the same direction as the TLCO, but is elevated when the lungs are normal but squashed or underinflated, for example in neuromuscular disease or scoliosis.

Blood gases

1. Oxygen. Arterial blood gases should always be interpreted in the light of the oxygen concentration that the patient was breathing at the time the sample was taken. This is particularly important when looking at the PaO_2. A low PaO_2 (or lower than expected for that inspired oxygen concentration) can be caused by inadequate ventilation of the alveoli, impaired diffusion, ventilation/perfusion imbalance or a right-to-left shunt.

2. Carbon dioxide. The $PaCO_2$ directly reflects the adequacy of alveolar ventilation. Hypoventilation causes a high $PaCO_2$ and hyperventilation a low $PaCO_2$. Inspection of the PaO_2 and acid-base status will usually indicate the cause of the abnormal $PaCO_2$.

3. Acid-base balance. The most common acid-base disturbance seen in respiratory patients is respiratory acidosis, that is an acidosis arising from an elevated $PaCO_2$. When this is present for more than a few hours, the bicarbonate level rises in an attempt to limit the effect of the $PaCO_2$ on pH.

Respiratory alkalosis is seen in patients hyperventilating (commonly either in an attempt to correct a low PaO_2, or on account of anxiety); in this case, after a few hours, compensatory mechanisms cause the bicarbonate concentration to fall, again in an attempt to minimize the effect on pH.

In a metabolic acidosis, the low pH is a potent stimulus to ventilation, and the hyperventilation which this produces leads to a fall in $PaCO_2$. The bicarbonate level is low on account of the metabolic disturbance.

Further Reading

Gibson GJ. *Clinical Tests of Respiratory Function.* London: Chapman and Hall, 1996.
Kinnear WJM. *Lung Function Tests – A Guide to their Interpretation.* Nottingham: Nottingham University Press, 1997.

Related topics of interest

MYCOBACTERIA

There are many species of mycobacteria, distributed widely through the environment. MTB is the comonest human pathogen. Other mycobacteria which may cause disease are called 'atypical mycobacteria', other terms for them being 'opportunistic', 'non-tuberculous' or 'environmental', and 'mycobacterium other than tuberculosis'.

Tuberculosis

1. Epidemiology. World-wide, one-third of the population are infected with MTB: annually 8 million develop TB, and 3 million die from it. In the UK, TB notification rates fell steadily (well before specific chemotherapy was available) until the late 1980s, since when there has been a modest increase. About 5000 cases of TB are notified annually in England and Wales at present.

Factors associated with the aquisition/reactivation of TB include immunocompromise (e.g. HIV, haematological malignancy, steroids), poverty, homelessness, alcoholism, diabetes mellitus and silicosis.

Immigrants from countries with a high TB incidence continue to have a higher risk of developing TB in the UK (e.g. the 1988 notification rate in Indian subcontinent patients was >100 per 10^5 compared with 5 per 10^5 in the indigenous white population). This increased risk applies also to children born in the UK of parents immigrating to the UK.

2. Natural history of infection. The only significant route of infection is by inhaling an aerosol containing MTB coughed up by patients suffering from pulmonary TB (almost always smear positive disease). In non-immune subjects (primary disease), organisms lodge in the alveoli and are taken up by macrophages with both local granulomatous consolidation, and transportation of bacilli to hilar and mediastinal glands.

In the lung, there may be local consolidation, usually in the mid- or lower-zones, segmental collapse owing to hilar node compression, bronchopneumonia owing to discharge of infection into the bronchial tree, and/or pleural effusion.

Blood stream dissemination occurs at this stage; foci of viable bacilli are more likely to survive in the upper part of the lungs, lymph nodes, kidney, brain and bone. Further spread and development is limited by development of cell-mediated immunity (as demonstrated by a positive tuberculin test within 4–10 weeks).

Up to 5% of recently infected individuals develop disease within a year. In others, the foci of infection heal or continue to contain viable bacilli which can later reactivate.

Reactivation (or post-primary) disease in the lung is characterized by an increased cellular response associated with specific immunity. Cavitation and fibrosis are marked in the upper zones.

3. Clinical features. Primary infection is usually asymptomatic (in >90% of patients). Symptoms in reactivated disease vary from none to rapidly progressive (consumption). Cough is common and may be highly productive, if cavitation occurs. In active disease haemoptysis occurs in about 8%. Fever and weight loss are not invariable. Pleuritic chest pain often accompanies effusion.

Signs are non-specific and may include consolidation, fibrosis and cervical nodes. Rarely, erythema nodosum occurs at the time of tuberculin conversion.

4. Investigations. The CXR in primary disease is abnormal in less than one-third of those with recent infection. The primary complex consists of a peripheral opacity (usually lower lobe) and hilar gland enlargement but bronchogenic spread, segmental or lobar collapse, miliary disease and pleural effusion may occur. The peripheral lesion may heal and calcify (a Ghon focus).

In reactivated disease, consolidation in the apical and/or posterior segments of the upper lobe or the apical lower lobe is common. Cavitation occurs in 40%. Fibrosis and calcification are common long-term sequelae. Old TB presents with a wide variety of CXR changes, and activity cannot be determined from the CXR.

Other presentations of TB include mediastinal gland enlargement on a CXR (especially in Asians), cervical glandular TB, pyrexia of unknown origin, and disease in other specific organs. TB in HIV-infected patients is discussed elsewhere.

Sputum examination with Ziehl–Nielson staining is vital. Three sputa should be sent to the laboratory. MTB may be present in sufficient quantity to be seen on sputum (termed smear positive, i.e. highly infectious) or if not, to grow in culture after 8–12 weeks. Nebulized saline is useful to obtain samples if sputum production is low. BAL at bronchoscopy is of proven value, especially when there is little or no sputum. A combination of sputum and BAL smear, and culture has greater than 90% sensitivity.

In a pleural effusion the pleural aspirate is smear positive in less than one-third but culture positive in more than two-thirds. Pleural biopsy adds to the diagnostic yield. Any tissue biopsies must be examined both histologically (for caseating granulomata) and sent fresh for culture. The yield from cervical gland aspiration is about 25% on smear, 50% on culture and greater than 90% when combined with histology.

Where samples are not obtainable, or have been negative despite a strong clinical suspicion, particularly with a PUO, a diagnostic trial of anti-tuberculous therapy is indicated. The role of tests based polymerase chain reaction amplification of mycobacterial DNA is currently confined to identification of organisms involved in epidemics, particularly of drug-resistant organisms. The tuberculin test (Heaf, Mantoux or Tine test is of limited value diagnostically. It can be helpful where there is known conversion from negative to positive, and where a positive test occurs before Bacille Calmette–Guérin (BCG) vaccination.

5. *Differential diagnosis.* The differential is extremely wide and includes:

- Other infections (e.g. atypical mycobacteria).
- Histoplasmosis, actinomycosis.
- Other causes of cavitation (e.g. cancer, vasculitis).
- Other causes of widespread nodular disease (e.g. sarcoidosis, CMV).
- Other causes of upper-zone disease (broncho-pulmonary aspergillosis, sarcoidosis, silicosis).
- Other causes of a mass and enlarged glands (e.g. carcinoma, lymphoma).

6. *Treatment.* It is vital to use standard drug regimes. In the UK there are regular updates on the management of TB from the Joint Tuberculosis Committee of the British Thoracic Society. A standard regime is rifampicin and isoniazid for 6 months with pyrazinamide and ethambutol in the first 2 months. These drugs all have high antibacterial activity and the cure rate with a fully sensitive organism approaches 100%. Minor adverse reactions occur in about 10% and major ones needing drug withdrawal in about 2%. Rifampicin, isoniazid and pyrazinamide can cause hepatotoxicity which may require at least temporary drug withdrawal in up to 5% of cases, usually in the early weeks of treatment. Pre-treatment liver function tests are recommended with regular monitoring if the patient has known chronic liver disease or initially raised tests. There is no need to monitor liver function tests otherwise. A rise in transaminase to more than five times normal mandates stopping anti-TB drugs.

Ethambutol can cause visual toxicity due to retrobulbar neuritis. Visual accuity should be tested at the outset and the patient warned to stop the drug if there are any visual effects. Ethambutol should be avoided in renal failure. It can be omitted in patients with a low risk of isoniazid resistance (e.g. previously untreated HIV negative patients).

In pregnancy, isoniazid, rifampicin, ethambutol, and probably pyrazinamide, are all safe. Streptomycin is absolutely contra-indicated owing to fetal ototoxicity.

Steroids may be beneficial in severely ill patients to improve symptoms. Studies have shown a reduced risk of developing constriction in pericarditis, but despite traditional teaching, steroids do not lessen residual pleural thickening after pleural effusion.

Drug resistance is a major problem in certain areas. In New York in the early 1990s, multi-drug resistance (MDR) occurred in more than one-third of cases. In the UK isoniazid resistance was reported in 1993 in approximately 3% of isolates and multi-drug resistance in less than 1%. MDR-TB has a poor prognosis. Management strategies include routinely using ethambutol in the initial regime, and using newer drugs, for example rifabutin, quinolones. Directly observed therapy (DOT), that is treatment supervized 2 or 3 times a week, has been particularly effective, resulting in a substantial reduction in MDR-TB.

7. *Outcome.* Relapse occurs in up to 3% after treatment. Long-term pulmonary consequences of TB include fibrosis, bronchiectasis (with associated haemoptysis) and colonization of old cavities by aspergillus.

8. *Control and prevention.* In the UK TB is a statutorily notifiable disease. Notification triggers appropriate contact tracing by the network of contact clinics. Contact tracing procedures are beyond the scope of the present text. Even smear positive patients become effectively non-infectious after 2 weeks of adequate drug therapy.

Hospital admission is required only on the grounds of severe illness, problems with TB drugs including compliance, and social reasons. Those with smear positive disease needing hospital admission should be in a single room for 2 weeks. There is no infective risk from linen, crockery etc.

The programme of BCG vaccination to all children aged 10–14 at school is continuing. BCG is 80% protective in the UK though elsewhere wide variation in protection has been reported. All health care workers should have a pre-employment screen with a tuberculin test where there is no BCG scar, and CXR depending on the tuberculin test and symptoms.

Chemoprophylaxis with isoniazid and rifampicin for 3 months is indicated for children or young adults with strongly positive Heaf tests who have not had BCG, or where there has been documented recent tuberculin test conversion. It is also considered for patients on long-term steroids or other immunosupressants where a CXR suggests previous untreated TB.

Tuberculosis and HIV

Patients with dual infection of MTB and HIV have an 8–10% annual progression to active TB, compared with 5–10% lifetime risk in those with a normal immune system. The CXR appearances are often atypical. The tuberculin test may be negative in active disease and sputum is more often negative. Other mycobacteria (e.g. *Mycobacterium avium intracellularae*) are more common.

Response to standard treatment is good but there is a higher incidence of side effects. Treatment should be followed by isoniazid prophylaxis. BCG is not recommended as it may cause disseminated disease. In the USA it is recommended that tuberculin-positive HIV patients receive isoniazid prophylaxis.

Atypical mycobacteria

Atypical mycobacteria cause four main types of disease: pulmonary, lymphadenopathy, soft tissue, and disseminated disease in immmuno-compromized patients.

Pulmonary disease is mainly due to *M. kansasii* (MK), *M. malmoense* (MM), *M. avium intracellulare* (MAI), and *M. xenopi* (MX). Disseminated disease is usually due to MAI, and almost always in HIV disease.

1. Epidemiology. The atypical mycobacteria are ubiquitous and often found in soil and tap water. In 1994, atypical mycobacteria accounted for 24% of all mycobacterial isolates in England and Wales compared with 5% in 1982. The increased proportion is due to both a real increase in isolation (especially MAI in HIV) and to reductions in MTB. In non-immuno-compromized patients, disease usually occurs in later life on a background of pre-existing lung disease, for example COPD or old tuberculous disease. Atypical mycobacteria are non-transmissible.

2. Clinical features. No clinical or CXR features distinguish disease resulting from atypical mycobacteria from tuberculosis.

3. Investigations. As atypical mycobacteria can occur as contaminants, strict diagnostic criteria are needed – usually three positive cultures in sputum or BAL (or an appropriate biopsy) with clinical and/or CXR abnormalities compatible with mycobacterial disease. MAI may be grown from blood cultures in HIV disease.

4. Management. Treatment is much more difficult and less successful than for MTB. *In vitro* sensitivity testing often does not parallel clinical response. Ethambutol and rifampicin are the cornerstones of therapy. Such treatment can be used alone for MK and MX but must be given for at least 9 months. Even then there is a relapse rate of 9%. Clarithromycin and ciprofloxacin have good activity and recommended treatment for MAI or MM now includes at least one of these with ethambutol and rifampicin for up to 2 years. Surgical treatment (e.g. lobectomy) is effective for localized disease and can be useful in a fit patient when there is a poor response to, or relapse from, therapy.

Further reading

Davies PDO. Infection with *Mycobacterium kansasii*. *Thorax*, 1994; **49:** 435–436.

Joint Tuberculosis Committee of the British Thoracic Society. Chemotherapy and management of tuberculosis in the United Kingdom: recommendations 1998. *Thorax*, 1998; **53:** 536–548.

Mycobacterium avium disease: progress at last. *American Journal of Respiratory Critical Care Medicine*, 1996; **153:** 1737–1738.

Related topics of interest

NEUROMUSCULAR DISORDERS

Several groups of muscles are important for the maintenance of normal respiration. Upper airway muscles maintain the patency of the pharynx and larynx. The muscles of inspiration comprise the diaphragm, parasternal intercostals and accessory muscles of the neck. Expiratory muscles provide little contribution to quiet respiration, but are recruited when ventilation is increased and during coughing.

An abnormality of any part of the complex link between the respiratory centres and the muscles themselves can impair the normal function of the respiratory muscles.

1. Brainstem. Congenital absence of respiratory drive is known as 'Ondine's curse'. Encephalitis, syringobulbia, multiple sclerosis and multi-system atrophy can be associated with acquired loss of respiratory drive. Patients with severe obesity often have poor respiratory drive, with a central as well as obstructive component to their hypoventilation.

2. Spinal cord. Trauma, tumours, syringomyelia and multiple sclerosis are examples of lesions which may involve the spinal cord. The effect of spinal cord lesions on respiration depends upon their site. High cervical cord lesions lead to complete paralysis of the respiratory muscles and dependence on assisted ventilation, whereas if the lesion is below C5 diaphragm function is preserved. Thoracic spinal cord lesions have little effect on respiration.

3. Motor neurone. Trauma, surgery (phrenic nerve palsy after cardiac or cervical surgery), motor neurone disease, spinal muscular atrophy, ascending polyneuropathy (Guillain–Barré), and Charcot–Marie–Tooth disease may all affect respiratory motor neurones. The effects are most marked when the phrenic nerves are involved.

Respiratory paralysis in poliomyelitis was a common cause of death until the introduction of vaccination. Patients who had the disease in the 1950s frequently present with ventilatory failure as a late complication many decades later. This may represent late changes in their remaining respiratory muscles as a consequence of the disease, or deteriorating function as a part of normal ageing which reaches a critical threshold when normal ventilation cannot be sustained. In patients with paraspinal muscle paralysis, progression of scoliosis may increase the work of breathing. Upper airway obstruction and central respiratory drive problems can also be seen in polio.

Neuralgic amyotrophy is a condition where brachial neuritis causes shoulder pain and phrenic nerve palsy. There may be associated shoulder girdle weakness, manifest as winging of the scapula. Shortness of breath develops over a few days, and is often provoked by lying flat or immersion in a bath or swimming pool. If both phrenic nerves are affected, orthopnoea may be sufficiently severe to require non-invasive ventilation at night. Recovery is slow, often taking several years.

4. Neuromuscular junction. Myasthenia gravis may occasionally present as breathlessness, and assisted ventilation is sometimes necessary if respiratory paralysis is severe. The Eaton–Lambert syndrome is a paraneoplastic syndrome which produces a similar clinical picture.

5. Myopathies and dystrophies. Almost any disease of muscles may involve the respiratory muscles. Limb girdle dystrophy, acid maltase deficiency and facio scapulo humeral dystrophy can all affect the diaphragm at a stage when limb muscle function is still well preserved, whereas in Duchenne and Becker muscular dystrophies respiratory failure usually only develops when the disease is in an advanced stage. Dystrophia myotonica causes abnormalities of central respiratory drive and respiratory muscle weakness. Dermatomyositis and polymyositis occasionally cause ventilatory failure.

Clinical features

The symptoms of respiratory muscle dysfunction depend upon which muscles are affected and how severely. Unilateral diaphragm paralysis is often asymptomatic, but can cause dyspnoea on exertion. Bilateral diaphragm paralysis (or severe weakness) causes orthopnoea and dyspnoea on exertion. Generalized respiratory muscle weakness causes breathlessness, but often initially manifests as nocturnal hypoventilation with sleep disturbance, morning headache and daytime sleepiness. Daytime respiratory failure develops at a later stage. Recurrent chest infections are seen in patients with a poor cough: normal inspiratory, expiratory, and upper airway muscle function are requisites for an effective cough. Bulbar muscle incoordination or weakness leads to aspiration pneumonia.

Management

With a few exceptions (myasthenia gravis or polymyositis, for example) it is seldom possible to treat the underlying neuromuscular disease. Regular monitoring of respiratory function, particularly vital capacity, is important to predict the onset of ventilatory failure. In diseases which may progress over a few hours, for example myasthenia gravis or Guillain–Barré, the patient should be transferred to an intensive care unit when the vital capacity falls to 1 l.

Hypercapnia is occasionally precipitated by a clearly identifiable factor, for example sedative drugs, but in most patients with neuromuscular disease it is a worrying development which requires prompt action. Once a patient is hypercapnic, they may get rapidly worse and are likely to require assisted ventilation in the long term. A decision must be made as to whether this is appropriate and, if so, what modality is indicated. This may be non-invasive, or require endotracheal intubation until the situation is under control. Phrenic nerve pacing can be used in patients with spinal cord lesions or localized damage to the phrenic nerves at a fairly high site. Assisted coughing devices are available for patients with severe expiratory muscle weakness.

Further reading

Shneerson J. *Disorders of Ventilation*. Oxford: Blackwell, 1988.

Related topic of interest

Non-invasive ventilation (p. 114)

NON-INVASIVE VENTILATION

The development of mechanical assistance to ventilation was driven by devastating epidemics of poliomyelitis in the first half of the twentieth century. The successful introduction of endotracheal intubation in the 1950s diverted attention away from less invasive techniques, but in recent years there has been a resurgence of interest, particularly in the use of positive pressure ventilation through a nasal mask (nasal intermittent positive pressure ventilation – NIPPV), on which this chapter will concentrate.

Advantages

The main advantages of NIPPV over more invasive techniques are:

- Sedation is not required, so it is easy to provide ventilatory support on an intermittent basis.
- Complications of an endotracheal tube are avoided.
- Intensive care facilities may not be needed, and the equipment required is less costly than that for ventilation through an endotracheal tube.

Disadvantages

The disadvantages are:

- The airway is not protected, so in an unconscious patient there is a danger of inhalation of gastric contents if they vomit.
- Excessive secretions may be easier to suction through an endotracheal tube or tracheostomy.
- Nasal pressure sores may develop and necessitate use of an alternative interface or a break from NIPPV.
- Gastric distension.

Indications

1. *Acute hypercapnic respiratory failure.* NIPPV works well in patients with neuromuscular or skeletal chest wall problems who become hypercapnic acutely, on the background of chronic ventilatory problems. It is being used increasingly to treat acute exacerbations of COPD, although firm evidence of efficacy is still lacking. It is particularly useful to allow supplementary oxygen to be administered to patients who become severely hypercapnic when breathing oxygen without ventilatory assistance. Some patients with acute hypercapnic respiratory failure from other causes, for example acute asthma, have been managed with NIPPV, but the role of this technique in these situations is not yet clear.

2. *Chronic hypercapnic respiratory failure.* Patients with slowly progressive neuromuscular disease who develop hypercapnia and nocturnal hypoventilation experience dramatic and sustained improvement on nocturnal NIPPV. It may also be appropriate to treat some patients with rapidly progressive neuromuscular disease with NIPPV, mainly when severe

orthopnoea is disrupting sleep. Patients with skeletal chest wall problems respond similarly to those with slowly progressive neuromuscular disease. Central hypoventilation is always worse at night, and indeed may only be apparent then. NIPPV at night usually causes complete resolution of daytime symptoms.

Contra-indications

Patients with Type 1 respiratory failure (hypoxia without hypercapnia) do not respond well to NIPPV. In acute respiratory failure, impaired consciousness, cardio-vascular instability or a non-functioning gastro-intestinal tract are contra-indications to the use of NIPPV. Difficulties with excessive secretions have already been mentioned. Pneumonia of sufficient severity to produce hypercapnic respiratory failure will require endotracheal intubation.

Nasal masks cannot be used on patients with facial trauma. Poor cooperation precludes the use of NIPPV in around 50% of patients with acute respiratory failure. Poor motivation, problems with the dexterity required to apply the mask and inadequate home support may create difficulties with NIPPV at home.

Ventilator modes

1. Volume cycled. These ventilators deliver the tidal volume to which they are set, irrespective of the resistance that the ventilator experiences. Ventilation will therefore be maintained if the patient changes position or becomes more difficult to ventilate for some other reason, for example accumulation of secretions in the bronchial tree. Since some air is inevitably lost through leaks during NIPPV, the ventilator tidal volume should be set at 1.5 times that which needs to be delivered to the lungs.

2. Pressure cycled. Pressure cycled (or pressure pre-set) ventilators will deliver a variable tidal volume, depending on the compliance of the respiratory system. Their main advantage for NIPPV is that they compensate for mask leakage.

3. Pressure support. These ventilators provide positive pressure from when the patient starts to breathe in until they start to exhale. The assistance to breathing they receive is more closely synchronized with their own respiratory cycle, so this technique is particularly valuable when the spontaneous pattern of breathing is variable. Bi-level positive airway pressure combines inspiratory pressure support with a lower expiratory positive pressure.

Patient interfaces

A nasal mask is suitable for most patients. A chin strap can be used to prevent the mouth falling open. A full face mask can be used, but is less comfortable. Nasal pillows are useful when a nasal mask has caused ulceration of skin over the bridge of the nose. Mouthpieces have been used long-term for patients with neuromuscular disease.

Monitoring

Measurement of blood gases after 30 min of NIPPV in patients with acute respiratory failure will indicate if the technique is likely to be succesful. Overnight oxygen saturation and day-time arterial blood gases will improve over several days. For patients commencing long-term nocturnal NIPPV, if overnight oximetry shows a mean saturation of less than 80% supplementary oxygen should be considered. Measurement of overnight transcutaneous carbon dioxide tension is not necessary provided the overnight saturation is satsifactory with the patient breathing air, but may be needed when oxygen is used.

Discharge

A home visit is desirable prior to discharge. The patient should be contacted regularly in the first few days at home, and reviewed in the clinic 2–3 weeks later. The interval between subsequent follow-up visits will vary with circumstances, but will usually be around 3 months. Overnight monitoring is only necessary if there is deterioration in the patient's condition, for example the development of right heart failure.

Further reading

Kinnear WJM. *Assisted Ventilation at Home*. Oxford: Oxford University Press, 1996.
Simmonds AK. *Non-invasive Respiratory Support*. London: Chapman and Hall, 1996.

Related topics of interest

Chronic obstructive pulmonary disease (p. 37)
Neuromuscular disorders (p. 111)
Skeletal disorders (p. 150)
Sleep apnoea (p. 152)

PLEURAL EFFUSION

Several litres of pleural fluid are produced each day by the parietal pleura in normal individuals, but the visceral pleura is able to absorb this volume easily and only a few millilitres remain in the pleural space at any one time.

When the production of fluid increases, either because of a high hydrostatic pressure or low oncotic pressure, the visceral pleura may not be able to cope with the additional volume and a pleural effusion accumulates. This form of effusion is called a transudate, which is a dilute effusion with a protein content less than 30 g/l and few cells. The pleural surfaces themselves are normal, but the dynamics of fluid transport across them have been disturbed.

When the visceral pleura is thickened, its ability to absorb fluid is impaired. Moreover, inflamed visceral or parietal pleura may exude high-protein fluid and cells. These are removed from the pleural space at a much slower rate through lymphatics. These factors result in the accumulation of fluid with a protein content greater than 30 g/l in the pleural space. Such effusions are called exudates.

Aetiology

1. Transudates. Cardiac failure usually causes bilateral effusions (although 50% of patients with bilateral effusions and a normal heart size on CXR will have malignant effusions). Unilateral effusions should only be ascribed to cardiac failure after investigations for other causes are negative. Classically, cardiogenic effusions are transudates. However, when the patient is taking high-dose diuretics, faster reabsorption of water than protein from the effusion can push the protein concentration above 30 g/l.

Hypoproteinaemia resulting, for example, from cirrhosis, the nephrotic syndrome, protein-losing enteropathy and severe malnutrition may also cause a transudate.

2. Exudates. Any pneumonia (including tuberculosis) can be associated with a pleural effusion, which may develop into an empyema. Cancer (lung cancer, breast cancer, mesothelioma) is a common cause of pleural effusion: 70% of massive effusions (>2l) are malignant in origin. RA and SLE cause exudative effusions. Small effusions may also be seen following pulmonary infarction.

Rarer causes of an exudate are intra-abdominal pathology (sub-phrenic abscess, viral hepatitis, hepatic abscess, pancreatitis), Sjogren's syndrome, Familial Mediterranean Fever, Wegener's granulomatosis, sarcoidosis, aortic dissection, oesophageal rupture, Dressler's syndrome, Meig's syndrome, uraemia, hypothyroidism, hyperthyroidism, benign asbestos disease and drugs (nitrofurantoin, dantrolene, methysergide, bromocryptine, procarbazine, methotrexate, practolol).

3. Haemothorax. Bleeding into the pleural space may be traumatic, iatrogenic (e.g. subclavian arterial puncture during central venous cannulation) or related to a bleeding diathesis.

Pleural endometriosis, pulmonary sequestration or rupture of an AV malformation may occasionally cause a haemothorax.

4. Chylothorax. Lipid accumulation is seen in any pleural effusion that has been present for many years (e.g. in rheumatoid arthritis), from breakdown of cells. Disruption of the thoracic duct by tumour, trauma or surgery will lead to a chylothorax. Other causes are left subclavian vein thrombosis, yellow nail syndrome, filariasis, cirrhosis, heart failure, aortic aneurysm, and lymphangioleiomyomatosis.

Clinical features

A small pleural effusion may be asymptomatic. Associated pleurisy may cause pain. Shortness of breath and cough develop with larger collections of pleural fluid. Clinical examination will only detect pleural collections of at least 500 ml. Diminished expansion, dull percussion, decreased tactile vocal fremitus and decreased breath sounds are the physical signs. Breath sounds may be increased at the top of the fluid (possibly over adjacent atelectatic lung). Mediastinal shift in large effusions will be reflected by the position of the trachea and apex beat. A large effusion without mediastinal shift suggests that the mediastinum is fixed (for example by malignant infiltration) or that there is collapse of part of the lung.

Investigations

Blunting of the costo-phrenic angle is the first radiographic sign of a pleural effusion on the CXR, but at least 200 ml of fluid must be present for this to be seen. In larger effusions a meniscus of fluid is seen extending up the chest wall, with complete opacification of the hemithorax in massive effusions. Large volumes of fluid (>1 l) can collect underneath the lung in a sub-pulmonary effusion. In this instance, the CXR appearances at first sight appear to be those of a raised hemidiaphragm; however, the apex of the shadow is more lateral and on the left the stomach bubble is not elevated. On a supine film a pleural effusion causes diffuse opacification. CT or ultrasound can be used to differentiate pleural fluid from thickening and identify loculation, and to look for liver and sub-phrenic abscesses.

The need for blood tests will be guided by the clinical scenario, but may include a full blood count, ESR, rheumatoid factor, anti-nuclear factor, urea, electrolytes, liver function tests, total protein, albumen, thyroid function tests and amylase. An electrocardiogram (ECG) and echocardiography should be performed if there is suspicion of heart failure.

Pleural aspiration is usually necessary to ascertain the aetiology. Specimens should be sent for:

- Protein to distinguish transudates from exudates.
- Microscopy and culture.

- Cytology (positive in 70% of malignant effusions).

Other measurements which can be of value are the pH (low in empyema), amylase if pancreatitis is suspected, and triglycerides if the fluid appears milky (chylothorax). Low glucose levels are seen in empyema and rheumatoid effusions. Lactate dehydrogenase levels can be used to differentiate transudates from exudates if the protein level is equivocal. Many other parameters have been measured in pleural fluid, but their clinical utility is poor.

If the cause is not revealed on a specimen of pleural fluid, pleural biopsy should be performed. Specimens should be sent in fixative for histology, and also in normal saline for mycobacterial culture. Tuberculosis of the pleural cavity is more commonly diagnosed on pleural biopsy specimens than on pleural fluid. Thoracoscopy will be necessary if no diagnosis is apparent from the above investigations.

Treatment

Treatment should be given for the underlying condition. Therapeutic aspiration of 1000–1500 ml (less if the patient starts to cough or experiences chest pain) will improve shortness of breath. Insertion of an intercostal drain allows removal of all the fluid in the pleural space, and may be followed by pleurodesis with tetracycline or talc for recurrent malignant effusions. Thoracic duct ligation is of value in chylothorax.

Further reading

Walshe ADP, Douglas JG, Kerr KM, McKean ME, Godden DJ. An audit of the clinical investigation of pleural effusion. *Thorax*, 1992; **47:** 734–737.

Related topics of interest

PNEUMOCONIOSIS

The term pneumoconiosis encompasses the effect of inhaled dust on the lung excluding the development of neoplasia or asthma. The effects of dusts can be classified as:

- Fibrogenic, for example asbestos, coal, silica.
- Non-fibrogenic, for example iron, tin, barium.
- Granulomatous, for example beryllium, organic dusts.

Asbestos and organic dusts causing extrinsic allergic alveolitis are covered in the relevant chapters. The development of harmful effects depends on whether dust particles are of an appropriate size (0.5–10 μm) to be deposited in the lung, and whether such dust is toxic to macrophages.

Coal workers pneumoconiosis (CWP)

Coal dust can cause:

- Simple CWP.
- Complicated CWP.
- Silicosis.
- Bronchitis.
- Emphysema.

The distinction between CWP and silicosis can be confusing. Coal contains varying quantities of quartz (i.e. silica). The CXR appearances of CWP and silicosis can be identical. However, coal dust certainly causes CWP even in the absence of silica. To complicate matters, silicosis can occur in coal workers who drill through rock (as opposed to coal) strata. Workers at the pit face have the highest coal dust exposure. However, even for this group, dust levels have greatly declined in recent years. Both simple and complicated CWP are defined by their CXR appearances, which are classified by the International Labour Organization (ILO) system, by comparison with standard films.

1. Simple CWP. Simple CWP is defined by small round opacities up to 10 mm in size on a CXR. These opacities represent accummulation of dust with some fibrosis and focal emphysema. The differential diagnosis of this CXR appearance is:

- Occupational causes, for example CWP, silicosis, siderosis, etc.
- EAA.
- Miliary tuberculosis.
- Sarcoidosis.
- Micrometastases.
- Haemosiderosis.
- Chicken pox pneumonia.

Simple CWP is not associated with symptoms, signs or reduced lung function. The occurrence and progression of CWP is related to cumulative dust exposure and number of years underground, but the extent of the CXR change is not related to FEV_1. It is now, however, accepted that coal dust exposure causes airways obstruction (emphysema) independently of both smoking and the CXR appearances.

2. Complicated CWP. Complicated CWP is also known as Progressive Massive Fibrosis (PMF) and is defined by large CXR opacities (>1 cm diameter), usually but not always on a background of simple CWP. Pathologically, the lesions of PMF are black masses of fibrosis and coal dust with surrounding emphysema. They frequently enlarge and may cavitate. PMF is associated with increasing breathlessness and productive cough with a mixed obstructive restrictive ventilatory defect.

3. Caplan's syndrome (also known as rheumatoid pneumoconiosis). This is the occurrence of multiple round CXR opacities in coal workers who have seropositive rheumatoid arthritis. The opacities have the histological features of rheumatoid nodules. Caplan's syndrome is usually asymptomatic and may precede joint disease.

Silicosis

Silicosis is due to the inhalation of the crystalline form of silicon dioxide (e.g. quartz). Occupations with a risk of silicosis include mining and tunnelling through hard rock, sand blasting or fettling in foundries, stone masons, or the ceramics industry. CXR opacities correspond to the silicotic nodule – formed from concentric layers of collagen surrounding a central aggregate of silica. Radiographically, rounded opacities develop, mainly in the mid- and upper-zones, sometimes with irregular fibrosis, and which may progress to PMF. There may be hilar gland enlargement and both the opacities and the glands may develop egg shell calcification.

With progressive CXR change there is gradually increasing breathlessness with impairment of ventilatory capacity and gas transfer. CXR progression is common after exposure ceases. No treatment is available. There is a greatly increased risk of tuberculosis: quartz is highly toxic to macrophages and their ability to kill mycobacteria. There is an association with systemic sclerosis and a possible increased risk of lung cancer. Acute silicosis resulting from massive exposure presents with rapid onset of breathlessness, crackles and CXR appearances of pulmonary oedema. It is rare but frequently fatal.

Other fibrogenic dusts

Talc, kaolin (china clay), mica, polyvinylchloride, and many other agents may cause pneumoconiosis. Man-made mineral fibres, such as glass fibre, do not appear to cause disease.

Inert (non-fibrogenic) dusts

These dusts do not cause fibrosis or other local toxicity. High radiodensity dusts show rounded opacities of varying size on CXR while other dusts may show no evidence of lung retention. Iron (siderosis), tin (stannosis), barium (baritosis), and antimony all cause opacities up to 2 mm in diameter on CXR of uniform distribution often with Kerley B lines and hilar lymphadenopathy. These dusts cause no symptoms or lung function impairment. The lesions usually fade after exposure ceases and there is no risk of lung cancer. Cement (main constituent limestone) and gypsum (used in plaster manufacture) are low radiodensity dusts, and not associated with CXR abnormalities or symptoms. However, workers may be exposed to quartz contamination of these dusts with resultant impairment.

Berylliosis

Beryllium use has been in metal alloys and in fluorescent lighting tube manufacture. Beryllium can cause a systemic granulomatous disease resembling sarcoidosis, with pulmonary fibrosis and increasing breathlessness. In contrast to sarcoidosis, peripheral lymphadenopathy and CNS or eye involvement do not occur. Steroids are helpful but resolution is rare. Host susceptibility is probably critical. The development of berylliosis is associated with HLA–DPB alleles with a glutamate residue at position 69 of the β chain.

Other dusts and fumes

Welders are at risk of several lung problems including siderosis, occupational asthma (e.g. isocyanates), bronchitis, and metal fume fever. Metal fume fever (welders or foundry workers are susceptible) gives flu-like symptoms occurring a few hours after exposure to various metal fumes (e.g. zinc, copper, magnesium). Tolerance develops but is lost after a short period away (e.g. a weekend, hence the term 'Monday morning fever'). Complete recovery occurs over 1–2 days.

Aluminium dust exposure may cause asthma (pot room workers are susceptible), or pulmonary fibrosis (similar to fibrosing alveolitis). Cadmium, used in corrosion-resistant alloys, causes renal dysfunction, acute pneumonitis and probably emphysema. Cobalt, used for its resistance to heat and wear in hard metal combinations with tungsten, causes acute pneumonitis, asthma and pulmonary fibrosis. Chromium, nickel and arsenic exposures lead to an increased risk of lung cancer.

Compensation

State compensation for pneumoconiosis is available in many countries. In the UK, a claimant is assessed by a Medical Board which decides whether pneumoconiosis is present and, if so, the attributable disability and pension. Civil action at common law is a further route to compensation.

Further reading

Morgan WKC, Seaton A. *Occupational Lung Diseases*. Philadelphia: WB Saunders, 1984.
Parkes WR. *Occupational Lung Disorders*. Oxford: Butterworth-Heinemann, 1994.

Related topic of interest

Asbestos (p. 5)

PNEUMONIA

Pneumonia is a common condition, with an incidence of 1–3 per 1000 of the adult population per year. Many cases are mild, with only 25% being admitted to hospital, but it is still an important cause of death in previously fit young adults. Over the age of 65 years, 6% of deaths are primarily caused by pneumonia, and many more develop bronchopneumonia in the terminal phase of other illnesses.

Aetiology

Classification may be based on the part of the lung affected ('lobar pneumonia') or the aetiological agent ('bacterial pneumonia') but, in practice, it is more useful to subdivide pneumonia by the place where the infection was contracted – the community or hospital.

1. Community-acquired pneumonia. Streptococcus pneumoniae is the commonest cause of pneumonia, accounting for up to 75% of cases. *Haemophilus influenzae* and *Moraxella catarrhalis* cause pneumonia mainly in patients with COPD. Secondary infection with *Staphylococcus aureus* during influenza epidemics is associated with high morbidity and mortality, especially in the elderly. *Klebsiella pneumoniae* also affects the elderly or debilitated patient, particularly chronic alcoholics. *Neisseria meningitides* may occasionally cause pneumonia.

Mycoplasma pneumoniae occurs in epidemics every 2–4 years, but is unusual in those over 60 years. It accounts for approximately 10% of cases of community-acquired pneumonia. *Chlamydia pneumoniae* is increasingly recognized as a cause of pneumonia. *Legionella pneumophila* may be contracted from water systems and *Chlamydia psittaci* from infected birds. *Coxiella burneti* (Q fever) occassionally causes small epidemics of pneumonia.

Influenza (A and B) and Parainfluenza viruses cause pneumonia. Varicella pneumonia is a complication of chicken pox with a high mortality.

Fungi are common pneumonic pathogens in immunocompromized patients, but in endemic areas coccidiodes, histoplasma and blastomycoses can cause a pneumonic illness in previously healthy individuals, varying from self-limiting mild episodes to life-threatening disease (usually with systemic dissemination).

2. Hospital-acquired pneumonia. Most of the agents which cause pneumonia in the community can do so in hospital. However, there are increased numbers of patients with gram negative infections. *Legionella pneumophila* persists in the water systems of many hospitals, and should always be considered in a patient who develops pneumonia during, or shortly after, a stay in hospital.

3. Pneumonia in the immuno-compromized host. The spectrum of pathogens causing pneumonia in this group of patients is much wider (see 'immunodeficiency').

4. Underlying lung disease. Patients with COPD and bronchiectasis frequently have exacerbations associated with pneumonia (see 'Chronic obstructive pulmonary disease' and 'Bronchiectasis').

Clinical features

Pneumonia is usually a febrile illness associated with rigors and sweating. Cough is often unproductive in the initial stages, with purulent secretions being expectorated a few days later. Blood may be mixed in with the sputum. Breathlessness and pleuritic chest pain are also common. Headache and myalgia are features of atypical infections (Mycoplasma, Chlamydia, etc), which are also characterized by a prodromal illness of 1 week or more, often with a sore throat and involvement of other members of the household. Abdominal pain may be the dominant symptom in lower lobe pneumonia, and careful respiratory assessment is important in the patient with an acute abdomen. This is particularly relevant when pneumonia is complicated by abnormal liver function and jaundice. Drowsiness and confusion can be present in any severe pneumonia, but are often seen in patients with Legionella infection.

Pyrexia is usual, but may be absent in the elderly. *Herpes labialis* can be seen in any pneumonia, not just pneumococcal. Central cyanosis is a feature of more severe infections. Hypotension suggests that the patient may be septicaemic and/or dehydrated. Tachypnoea is an important pointer to the presence of a severe pneumonia (see below). Dullness to percussion, increased tactile vocal fremitus and bronchial breathing are heard over a consolidated lobe, together with coarse inspiratory crackles.

Investigations

The hallmark of pneumonia is the development of new radiographic shadowing in the lung fields. This may conform to the classical lobar distribution, but is usually patchy in atypical infections or bronchopneumonia. Associated pleural effusions are common. The differential diagnosis of the CXR appearances includes:

- Pulmonary oedema (which may occasionally be unilateral).
- Pulmonary infarction, either as a result of pulmonary embolism or vasculitis.
- Eosinophilic pneumonia. This is usually, but not always, associated with elevation of the blood eosinophil count,

but a mild eosinophilia may be seen in mycoplasma pneumonia.

- Non-infectious inflammation or fibrosis: pulmonary haemorrhage, organizing pneumonitis, FA, extrinsic allergic bronchioloalveolitis, and sarcoidosis may mimic pneumonia.

A full blood count, urea, electrolytes, liver function tests and blood cultures should be taken in all patients admitted to hospital with pneumonia. Oxygen saturation should also be measured in all patients, proceeding to arterial blood gases if it is less than 92%.

If the patient is producing sputum, it should be sent for microscopy and culture. (Gentle physiotherapy may be employed to help obtain a sputum sample, but more vigorous expectoration techniques should be used with great caution, since they may worsen gas exchange.) Bacterial antigens (*Pneumococcus*, *Legionella*, *Chlamydia*) may also be detected in the sputum, or in blood or urine. If present, pleural fluid should also be sampled and sent for microscopy, culture and bacterial antigens. An ultrasound or CT scan may help identify the optimal site to aspirate a parapneumonic effusion.

Serology for atypical infection is seldom helpful during the acute illness, but in combination with a convalescent sample helps identify the aetiological agent retrospectively. Bronchoscopy is indicated if there is suspicion of central obstruction lesion, for example a cancer or foreign body. BAL is important in identification of the infectious agent in immunocompromized patients, and is almost invariably performed in patients who need endotracheal intubation. Percutaneous needle biopsy and open lung biopsy have also been used to determine the aetiology of pneumonia, but are not in common usage.

Assessment of severity

1. *Major risk factors.*

- Respiratory rate greater than 30 breaths/min.
- Urea greater than 7 mmol/l.
- Diastolic blood pressure less than 60 mm Hg.

The presence of two or more of these is associated with a greatly increased risk of death, and indicates the need for close monitoring in an intensive care or high dependancy unit.

2. *Other risk factors.*

- Age more than 60 years.
- Underlying disease.
- Multilobar involvement.
- Hypoalbuminaemia.
- Confusion.

- White blood cell count less than 4 or greater than $20 \times 10^9/l$.
- Bacteraemia.
- Atrial fibrillation.
- Arterial PaO_2 less than 8 kPa.

Complications

Pleural effusion occurs in 40% of patients. This may be sterile, or become infected (see 'Empyema'). Abscess formation (see 'Lung abscess') is associated with persistent fever cavitation, which should be distinguished from a pneumatocoele, which is a sterile air-filled space following a necrotizing pneumonia. Metastatic abscesses may also develop.

Abnormal renal and hepatic function can occur in any pneumonia, but are common in Legionella infections. Erythema multiforme, arthritis and haemolysis suggest myscoplasma infection. Endocarditis can complicate coxiella infection. Dactylitis is a rare feature of pneumococcal speticaemia. Pneumonia may precipitate heart failure, particularly in elderly patients. ARDS may develop in severe cases of pneumonia.

Treatment

Oxygen should be administered if the oxygen saturation is less than 92%, usually in high concentration since carbon dioxide retention in pneumonia is extremely rare unless there is underlying lung disease. Intravenous fluid will usually be necessary on account of increased insensible water loss (pyrexia and mouth breathing) and vasodilatation.

Initial antibiotic therapy should be guided by the severity of the illness and the setting in which it occurs:

- Amoxycillin 500 mg PO tds is adequate for mild cases, or erythromycin 500 mg qds PO for patients who are allergic to penicillin.
- Ampicillin 500 mg qds IV together with erythromycin 500 mg qds PO should be given to moderately severe cases (cefuroxime 1.5 g tds IV instead of ampicillin if allergic).
- Severe cases will need a cephalosporin such as cefuroxime 1.5 g tds IV together with clarithromycin 500 mg bd IV.
- Hospital-acquired pneumonia has conventionally been treated with a cephalosporin such as cefuroxime 1.5 g tds IV, but the widespread use of cephalosporins for pneumonia may promote outbreaks of Clostridium difficile diarrhoea. Benzyl penicillin 1.2 g qds IV, together with ofloxacin 400 mg bd PO, is an alternative combination which is less likely to cause such problems. Newer quinolone antibiotics may prove to be adequate as monotherapy for community-acquired pneumonia.

Antibiotics should be given for at least 3 days after fever settles or 7 days, whichever is longer. The choice of antibiotics may be changed when culture and sensitivity results become available. Although antibiotic resistance of Pneumococci (and some other organisms causing pneumonia) is a worrying development, resistance is only partial and, provided adequate doses are used, there is as yet no cause to change the above recommendations.

Outcome
The overall mortality of community-acquired pneumonia is around 5%, but 20% for those admitted to hospital and 50% if intensive care is required.

Further reading

British Thoracic Society guidelines for the management of community acquired pneumonia in adults admitted to hospital. *British Journal of Hospital Medicine*, 1993; **49:** 346–350.
Godfrey S, Wilson R. *Pneumonia*. London: Martin Dunitz, 1996.
Torres A, Woodhead M. eds. *Pneumonia*, European Respiratory Monograph, Volume 2 Number 3, 1997.

Related topics of interest

PNEUMOTHORAX

The incidence of spontaneous pneumothorax is around 10 per 100 000 of the adult population per year. It is more common in males and tall people, and occasionally runs in families.

Aetiology

1. Primary. Spontaneous in the absence of an underlying cause.

2. Traumatic. For example, after a stab injury or rib fracture.

3. Iatrogenic. After percutaneous lung biopsy, intercostal nerve block, central venous cannulation or pleural biopsy.

4. Secondary. Associated with underlying lung disease:

- Emphysema, COPD, asthma.
- CF.
- FA.
- Cavitating pneumonia or other cavitating/cystic lung disease (such as pulmonary infarction, neurofibromatosis, Langerhan's cell histiocytosis, lymphangioleiomyomatosis, etc.).
- Connective tissue disease (Ehlers–Danlos and Marfan's syndromes).

Clinical features

Small pneumothoraces are often asymptomatic. Shortness of breath occurs in larger pneumothoraces or with a smaller pneumothorax if there is underlying lung disease. Chest pain is common and may be sharp or dull in character. Air may be palpable in the subcutaneous tissues (subcutaneous emphysema) or cause visible swelling in the neck or around the eyes. The chest is hyperinflated on the side of the pneumothorax, with reduced expansion, a hyper-resonant percussion note, and diminished breath sounds. Clicks or crunches in time with cardiac systole may be audible.

A tension pneumothorax is defined by the presence of circulatory collapse, with tachycardia and hypotension. Mediastinal shift is indicated by deviation of the trachea or apex beat, but is not synonymous with tension.

Investigations

The CXR reveals a line corresponding to the visceral, with no lung markings peripheral to this line. The CXR should be taken on inspiration, with no additional information provided by an expiratory film. In a severely ill patient, for example in the intensive care unit, it may only be possible to obtain a supine film, on which the appearances of a pneumothorax are darkness with depression of the hemidiaphragm, since the air occupies an anterior position. CT scanning easily detects a pneumothorax in cases of doubt, and may also show underlying lung disease.

Oxygen saturation should be measured in any patient with a pneumothorax who is breathless or cyanosed. Arterial blood gases are seldom necessary, since carbon dioxide retention is unusual unless there is underlying lung disease or the patient is in extremis with bilateral pneumothoraces.

Management

Observation is all that is needed in a patient with normal lungs who is not breathless and with only partial collapse of the lung on the CXR. In spontaneous pneumothorax, aspiration should be performed before resorting to insertion of an intercostal drain. Indications for aspiration are as follows:

- Any patient with a pneumothorax who is breathless.
- Complete collapse of the lung.
- Moderate collapse in a patient with underlying lung disease.

Aspiration should be performed in the second intercostal space (ICS) anteriorly in the mid-clavicular line, or in the axilla. After instillation of 10–20 ml of 1% lignocaine, an intravenous cannula is inserted into the pneumothorax and the inner metal part removed. Using a 50 ml syringe and three-way tap, 2500 ml are removed (or less if patient starts to cough). Overnight observation is only necessary afterwards if there is underlying lung disease.

An intercostal drain should be inserted in all patients with traumatic and tension pneumothoraces, or if aspiration has not reduced the size of the pneumothorax. The fouth, fifth or sixth ICS in the mid-axillary line above the level of the nipple is the safest region for insertion of a drain. After instillation of 20 ml of 1% lignocaine, a skin incision 1–2 cm wide is made using a number 11 blade. Blunt dissection down to the parietal pleura then makes a track wide enough for the drain. A 20–24 F drain is inserted without force a short distance into the pleural cavity, the trocar directed up to the apex of the lung, and the drain advanced off the trocar until only 5 cm remains outside the chest. The trocar is then removed and the drain attached to an underwater seal or flutter valve. The drain is sutured in place using a strong suture – a purse string suture for closing the wound should be done at the time of removal of the drain rather than at insertion.

Suction should be applied if air is still bubbling through the underwater seal or flutter valve the next day. The drain can be removed 24 h after bubbling has ceased, provided the CXR shows full expansion of the lung.

Surgical intervention, usually thoracoscopic, is needed if an air leak persists after 7 days. Chemical pleurodesis should be considered for a persistent air leak or recurrent pneumothorax in a patient who is not fit for surgical pleurodesis.

Outcome	After a single pneumothorax, about 30% of patients have a recurrence within 5 years, or 50% after a second pneumothorax. Therefore, surgical pleurodesis is recommended after a second pneumothorax.

Further Reading

Miller AC, Harvey JE. Guidelines for the management of spontaneous pneumothorax. *British Medical Journal*, 1993; **307:** 114–116.

Related topics of interest

Asthma (p. 17)
Chronic obstructive pulmonary disease (p. 37)
Cystic fibrosis (p. 52)
Diffuse parenchymal lung disease (p. 59)
Emphysema (p. 69)
Pneumonia (p. 124)

PREGNANCY

Most pregnant women have mild exertional breathlessness in the late stages of pregnancy. The main difficulty in assessing patients with respiratory symptoms during pregnancy is distinguishing between the normal physiological response to pregnancy, the effect of pregnancy on pre-existing cardiorespiratory disease and true pregnancy-related cardiorespiratory disease.

Physiological response to pregnancy

The main physiological responses to pregnancy include:

- Increased circulating blood volume and cardiac output.
- Decreased FRC + RV.
- Increased minute ventilation (believed to be due to elevated progesterone levels).
- Compensated respiratory alkalosis.

Respiratory conditions in pregnancy

1. Asthma. Asthma may improve, remain the same, or deteriorate during pregnancy. Approximately one-third of pregnant asthmatics fall into each of these categories. However, individuals whose asthma deteriorates markedly during pregnancy often have problems in subsequent pregnancies. A small number of patients may present with asthma during pregnancy: this can be difficult to distinguish from pregnancy-related hyperventilation.

2. Pulmonary embolism. The risk of thromboembolic disease increases during pregnancy. With the increasing recognition of genetic defects causing thrombophilia, such patients will require full assessment postnatally. The diagnosis of pulmonary emboli poses practical problems. Although the radiation exposure of the foetus during a CXR is extremely small, CXR should only be performed if the findings would potentially alter medical management. V/Q scans also carry a minimal theoretical risk to the foetus, but again should be reserved for situations where the result of the scan will alter patient management. One option is to perform a perfusion scan alone unless there is a good reason for requiring a ventilation scan as well, for example where there is other underlying lung disease. Lower limb doppler studies are safe in pregnancy. Treatment also causes difficulties: warfarin is teratogenic and should be avoided in the first trimester, so proven pulmonary emboli have to be treated with an extended course of heparin.

3. Cardiac disease. An important cause of worsening breathlessness during pregnancy is previously unrecognized cardiac disease, for example mitral stenosis resulting from previous rheumatic fever. Pregnancy can also produce a cardiomyopathy, although this is very rare. Finally, severe anaemia may worsen pregnancy-related dyspnoea.

Further reading

Rizk NW, Kalassian KG, Gilligan T, Druzin MI, Daniel DL. Obstetric complications in pulmonary and critical care medicine. *Chest*, 1996; **110:** 791–809.

Related topics of interest

PULMONARY EMBOLISM

Acute pulmonary embolism is a potentially life-threatening but treatable medical emergency. The diagnosis is often only established post-mortem, pulmonary embolism being a frequent terminal event in patients with other disease. At the other end of the spectrum, patients with suspected pulmonary embolism are responsible for a substantial part of the acute medical work load of the average district general hospital.

Aetiology

Pulmonary embolism is usually due to thrombus arising in the venous circulation embolizing to the pulmonary arterial circulation. Although the site of origin is most frequently the deep veins of the calf, many other sources have been reported. Thrombus can arise *in situ* in the lung, giving rise to a picture similar to pulmonary embolism: this mechanism is probably important in sickling crises seen in patients with sickle cell anaemia. In addition, pulmonary embolism with infected thrombus (septic emboli, most frequently arising from endocarditis on the right-sided heart valves), air bubbles, or any particulate matter administered into the venous circulation (e.g. partially dissolved tablets in intravenous drug abusers) may present with similar symptoms.

Predisposing conditions

Many conditions potentially predisposing to stasis, vessel wall abnormality, or clotting disorders can lead to the development of thromboembolic disease:

- Immobility.
- Surgery/trauma to the lower limbs.
- Underlying neoplasia.
- Thrombophilia (e.g. antithrombin III deficiency).
- Oral contraceptive pill use.
- Severe intercurrent illness.
- Local immobilization (e.g. plaster cast).
- Smoking.
- Hormone replacement therapy.

Clinical features

1. Massive pulmonary embolism. Massive pulmonary embolus presents with cardiovascular collapse: the diagnosis should be suspected in anyone with acute onset of severe dyspnoea, hypotension and tachycardia with cyanosis. Signs of acute right ventricular strain may be present.

2. Small emboli. The signs of a small pulmonary embolus depend upon the actual size of the embolus. Very small emboli (lodging in sub-segmental pulmonary arteries) may produce no signs. At an early stage following an embolus the only abnormalities may be dyspnoea (which may not be apparent at rest), though some patients will have evidence of a degree of right ventricular strain with an elevated jugular venous pulse and a resting tachycardia. There may be evidence of a potential embolic source (deep venous thrombosis). A pleural rub may be audible. At a later stage, evidence of infarction may predominate (pleuritic pain, haemoptysis and dyspnoea).

Investigations

The ECG usually shows tachycardia with, in more severe cases, evidence of right ventricular strain giving rise to the classic $S_1 Q_3 T_3$ configuration. Right axis deviation, right bundle branch block and arrythmias (e.g. atrial fibrillation) may also be seen. CXR may be normal or may show an area of relative translucency. At a later stage, pulmonary infarction may be evident with often wedge-shaped areas of shadowing, which may cavitate, or linear atelectasis. Associated pleural effusions (small) are frequent.

Hypoxia (owing to ventilation perfusion mismatch) is a cardinal finding in pulmonary embolism: the diagnosis of significant pulmonary embolism is unlikely in the absence of hypoxia. The $PaCO_2$ may be low (owing to hyperventilation), normal, or high (in more severe disease).

V/Q scanning remains the most common diagnostic investigation in most UK hospitals. The result of the scan must be interpreted in the light of clinical information about the patient. Most centres report scans as normal, low, intermediate, or high probability. A normal scan is associated with an extremely low probability of pulmonary embolic disease and a high probability scan with greater than 80% likelihood of pulmonary embolic disease. The predictive value of low and intermediate probability scans are related to the associated clinical information. V/Q mismatch can be seen in other lung diseases, in particular in acute asthma and in chronic lung disease. In cases of doubt pulmonary angiography is helpful.

Pulmonary angiography remains the gold standard investigation, although its availability (particularly out of hours) is highly dependent on local services. Pulmonary angiography may be useful in the few patients with large pulmonary emboli in whom either thrombolytic therapy (which can be performed at the time of angiography) or embolectomy is contemplated.

If available, transthoracic echocardiography is a useful test which can demonstrate large central pulmonary emboli. The British Thoracic Society recommendations suggest that this should be the first test in a patient suspected of having a large pulmonary embolus. If the test is negative, further investigations should be performed.

Spiral CT is another promising technique for detecting clots in large pulmonary arteries. Magnetic resonance imaging (MRI) can be used to image the lungs and peripheral veins, easily detecting large and small pulmonary emboli and their source.

Management

Treatment of known pulmonary embolic disease should consist of a minimum of heparinization with either intravenous or subcutaneous low molecular weight heparin for at least 5 days. Oxygen should be administered whilst the patient remains hypoxic. Hypotension should be managed by central venous pressure monitoring, intravenous fluids to maintain a high central pressure, and inotropic support.

Proven acute massive pulmonary embolism should be treated with thrombolytic agents, either streptokinase or rTPA. The latter is less likely to cause systemic reactions. It can be administered through a peripheral vein. The dose is 100 mg over 2 h, followed by heparin when the activated partial prothrombin time falls to less than twice normal.

If a cardiothoracic surgeon is available on site, embolectomy can be performed and may be life-saving in some individuals. However, the time taken to organize acute embolectomy often precludes its use in those who would most benefit. The value of embolectomy in patients with more minor pulmonary emboli is limited.

Warfarin should be commenced within a few days, to overlap with heparin so that the patient receives at least 5 days of heparin. Warfarin should be continued for 3 months, unless risk factors or recurrent episodes indicate life-long treatment.

Outcome

Most patients with isolated small pulmonary emboli, for example secondary to immobilization resulting from a fracture, do well and have no long-term sequelae. The prognosis from acute massive pulmonary embolism is less good: even if immediate management is successful, these patients may subsequently develop pulmonary hypertension and be limited by breathlessness and right ventricular failure. Patients with more than one episode of thromboembolic disease, or with other risk factors, should be treated with long-term anticoagulation.

Further reading

Suspected acute pulmonary embolism: a practical approach. *Thorax*, 1997; **52:** Supplement 4.

Related topic of interest

Pulmonary hypertension (p. 139)

PULMONARY EOSINOPHILIA

Increased eosinophils in the lung tissue or airways can be caused by a variety of important respiratory conditions:

- Asthma.
- Pulmonary vasculitis (i.e. Churg Strauss syndrome).
- Acute eosinophilic pneumonia.
- Chronic eosinophilic pneumonia.
- Tropical pulmonary eosinophilia.

Asthma and pulmonary vasculitis are dealt with elsewhere. The other causes are discussed below.

Acute eosinophilic pneumonia

This is a condition of unknown aetiology which may either present acutely (acute eosinophilic pneumonia) or progress to chronic changes (chronic eosinophilic pneumonia).

1. Clinical features. The clinical features of acute eosinophilic pneumonia are those of an acute febrile illness accompanied by non-productive cough, dyspnoea, myalgia and, frequently, pleuritic chest pain. Crackles or wheeze may be heard on auscultation.

2. Investigations. The CXR shows segmental infiltrates: HRCT scanning often shows areas of ground-glass shadowing. Pleural effusions also occur frequently. Pulmonary function tests show a restrictive lung defect with reduced gas transfer. There is usually no peripheral eosinophilia at presentation although this may occur later in the disease. BAL shows marked eosinophilia.

3. Management. Patients with acute eosinophilic pneumonia usually respond to prednisolone (30–40 mg/day): following the resolution of radiological abnormalities steroids can usually be discontinued.

Chronic eosinophilic pneumonia

Patients with chronic eosinophilic pneumonia present with chronic symptoms suggestive of recurrent infection and/or asthma. Classic radiological abnormalities of bilateral peripheral infiltrates (with hilar sparing) may suggest the diagnosis. Other features include peripheral eosinophilia and BAL eosinophilia. The condition can be distinguished from Churg–Strauss syndrome by the absence of other systems involvement and the lack of vasculitic changes on biopsy. Treatment is with steroids but the response is far less good than in acute eosinophilic pneumonia.

Tropical pulmonary eosinophilia (TPE)

TPE is a condition with pulmonary clinical features similar to acute eosinophilic pneumonia which occurs in patients with parasitic (particularly GI) infection. The CXR usually shows perihilar infiltrates and there is invariably a marked peripheral eosinophilia. Treatment with anti-parasitic agents usually produces resolution of pulmonary symptoms, although these may recur with recurrent parasite exposure.

Further reading

Allen JN, Davis WB. Eosinophilic lung disease. *American Journal of Respiratory Critical Care Medicine*, 1994; **150:** 1423–1428.

Ong RKC, Doyle RL. Tropical pulmonary eosinophilia. *Chest*, 1998; **113:** 1673–1679.

Related topics of interest

Asthma (p. 17)
Diffuse parenchymal lung disease (p. 59)
Vasculitis (p. 163)

PULMONARY HYPERTENSION

Pulmonary hypertension may be of unknown cause (primary pulmonary hypertension) or secondary to cardiovascular disease (mitral stenosis, atrial septal defect), chronic hypoxia of any cause, drugs or recurrent pulmonary emboli.

Primary pulmonary hypertension (PPH)

PPH is a disease of unknown aetiology characterized by pulmonary hypertension in the absence of an underlying cause. Approximately 10% of cases are familial, suggesting that genetic factors are important in the development of the disease. Progressive pulmonary hypertension with features overlapping those seen in patients with PPH also occurs in a small number of patients who have taken anti-obesity drugs (fenfluramine and dexfenfluramine), chronic cocaine users, and HIV-positive patients (even in the absence of AIDS).

1. Clinical features. PPH is most common in women in the fourth to sixth decades. The presenting symptom is increasing exertional dyspnoea. Depending on the severity of pulmonary hypertension the clinical signs of right ventricular hypertrophy and/or failure may be present. These are:

- Right ventricular heave.
- Loud pulmonary component to the second heart sound.
- Elevated jugular venous pressure with prominent atrial and ventricular waves.
- Tricuspid regurgitation.
- Right ventricular third heart sound.
- Right heart failure.

2. Investigations. The diagnosis of PPH is one of exclusion. There are no specific features either on diagnostic tests or on histological examination. Investigations are aimed at excluding a secondary cause for pulmonary hypertension (see below).

3. Management. There are few controlled trials of treatments for PPH. Those studies which have been performed have tended to use surrogate end points (e.g. change in pulmonary artery pressure) rather than clinically relevant end points. Approximately 25% of patients show a haemodynamic response to vasodilators (e.g. calcium channel antagonists such as nifedipine). In selected patients, continuous ambulatory infusion of prostacyclin may be the treatment of choice. ACE inhibitors have been shown to produce haemodynamic improvement. Inhaled nitric oxide is also under investigation as a potential vasodilator in these patients. Patients with PPH are at increased risk for intrapulmonary thrombosis and hence should be treated with warfarin. Both lung and heart/lung transplantation are used in PPH. PPH has not been reported to recur following lung transplantation, although there is some evidence that obliterative bronchiolitis may be more common in these patients.

4. Outcome. Patients presenting with severe pulmonary hypertension (i.e. associated with evidence of right ventricular failure) have a poor prognosis with a mean survival of around 1 year. Patients with less severe disease obviously have a better prognosis: such patients should also be considered for lung transplantation.

Secondary pulmonary hypertension

1. Aetiology. Causes include chronic respiratory disease (e.g. COPD, CF, CFA, etc.), cardiac disease (mitral stenosis, atrial septal defect), recurrent pulmonary emboli, and systemic sclerosis.

2. Clinical features. The usual presentation is insidious onset of breathlessness although episodes of acute pulmonary emboli may be identified. The clinical signs of secondary PPH are indistinguishable from primary pulmonary hypertension (see above) unless there is evidence of the underlying cause. Particular attention should be paid to examining for underlying chronic respiratory or cardiac disease. Recurrent pulmonary emboli must be bilateral and extensive for pulmonary hypertension to develop.

3. Investigations. Arterial blood gases will show hypoxia. The CXR may show large pulmonary arteries and a prominent right ventricle. On HRCT there may be evidence of underlying lung diseases, if present. Ventilation perfusion scan may show multiple mismatched defects (e.g. in recurrent pulmonary emboli). Lung function tests in the absence of underlying respiratory disease will show normal lung volumes but reduced gas transfer. Cardiac catheterization and pulmonary angiography will show evidence of underlying cardiac disease, if present, and may reveal evidence of pulmonary embolic disease. MR angiography may prove useful, particularly in patients with suspected pulmonary emboli.

4. Management. Treatment is dependent upon underlying cause. If the underlying cause is irreversible, long-term oxygen therapy may be the only available option.

Further reading

Weir EK, Schremmer B. Vasodilators in the treatment of primary pulmonary hypertension. *European Respiratory Journal*, 1998; **12:** 263–264.

Related topic of interest

Pulmonary embolism (p. 134)

RENAL DISORDERS

Renal disease can be associated with lung problems in a number of ways. Firstly, many systemic diseases affect both organs, including:

- Sarcoidosis.
- Tuberculosis.
- Systemic vasculitis.
- Collagen-vascular disease, for example SLE.

Secondly, renal diseases can be associated with respiratory complications:

- Chronic renal failure: pneumonia, circulatory overload.
- Renal transplantation: pneumonia, drugs.
- Hypernephroma: metastases.
- Goodpasture's syndrome: pulmonary haemorrhage.

Thirdly, lung disease can be associated with renal complications, for example glomerulonephritis (especially membranoproliferative) as a non-metastatic complication of pulmonary malignancy. Some drugs used in the treatment of respiratory disease can cause or worsen renal failure (e.g. aminoglycoside antibiotics).

Goodpasture's syndrome

Goodpasture's syndrome is caused by circulating antibodies directed to antigens on the glomerular basement membrane (GBM). The condition presents with both renal and pulmonary manifestations. Autoantibodies are directed against epitopes on the alphaβ chain of type IV collagen, and probably other basement membrane epitopes.

1. Clinical features. Goodpasture's disease presents as a rapidly progressive glomerulonephritis with diffuse alveolar haemorrhage if the lung is also affected. Pulmonary involvement is much more common in patients with previous lung injury (e.g. from smoking) and there is evidence for genetic susceptibility from studies looking at major histocompatibility complex determinants: individuals with DR4 and DRw15 are at increased risk of developing Goodpasture's syndrome.

2. Pulmonary manifestations. In addition to the rapidly progressive glomerulonephritis (with red cells, white cells, casts and protein in the urine) and progressive acute renal impairment, patients with pulmonary disease usually present with worsening breathlessness, pulmonary infiltrates on CXR and haemoptysis.

3. Investigations. The diagnosis of Goodpasture's syndrome requires the demonstration of anti-glomerular basement membrane (anti-GBM) antibodies in serum or renal biopsy. About one-third of patients have negative serum anti-GBM antibodies but a diagnostic renal biopsy. One-fifth of patients with Goodpasture's syndrome also test positive for anti-neutrophil cytoplasmic antibodies (ANCA). The CXR in patients with pulmonary involvement shows diffuse pulmonary infiltrates: where significant haemorrhage occurs these may be rapidly progressive. Patients with marked pulmonary haemorrhage may be anaemic, and may have an increased transfer factor on lung function testing.

4. Management. Treatment consists of immunosuppression and renal replacement therapy if indicated.

Further reading

Pulmonary complications of systemic disease. In: Murray JF, ed. *Lung Biology in Health and Disease*, vol 59. Marcel Dekker, New York, 1992.
Kline Bolton W. Goodpasture's syndrome *Kidney International*, 1996; **50:** 1753–1766.

Related topics of interest

Drug-induced lung disease (p. 66)
Immunodeficiency (p. 90)
Sarcoidosis (p. 147)
Vasculitis (p. 163)

RHEUMATOLOGICAL DISORDERS

Most of the respiratory complications of 'rheumatological' disorders reflect their multi-system nature, although a more direct link is sometimes seen, for example costo-vertebral anklosis in ankylosing spondylitis.

RA

Respiratory complications of RA are usually seen in patients with florid joint disease, although, rarely, a lesion such as a pulmonary rheumatoid nodule may be the first manifestation of the disease. Fibrosing alveolitis in patients with RA is clinically and radiologically indistinguishable from CFA; in some patients the pattern of lung function test abnormality is different in that residual volume is elevated, or less severely reduced, than in the typical restrictive pattern of CFA, reflecting small-airway disease. The treatment of FA in rheumatoid patients is the same as for CFA. Very rarely, RA may be associated with upper lobe fibrosis similar to that seen in ankylosing spondylitis. Organizing pneumonitis has also been described.

Bronchiolitis obliterans in RA presents as breathlessness, with normal lung fields on the CXR. Lung function tests show elevation of residual volume and total lung capacity, with impaired gas transfer. Inflammation of bronchi in RA initially leads to a chronic productive cough. Bronchial wall damage subsequently produces the typical picture of bronchiectasis, which should be treated as for any other cause. Up to 20% of patients with RA have symptoms owing to pleural involvement. Small effusions are the commonest manifestation and occur more frequently in men. The fluid is usually an exudate with a low glucose concentration. Secondary infection may occur. Pulmonary rheumatoid nodules correspond to the lesions classically seen subcutaneously over the elbow. They may cavitate. In Caplan's syndrome, multiple small nodules occur in patients with coal-worker's pneumoconiosis and RA.

Several drugs used in the treatment of RA may cause lung disease, for example methotrexate, gold and sulphasalzine.

SLE

Pleurisy is the commonest pulmonary manifestation of SLE, often accompanied by a small exudative effusion. The disease also causes pneumonitis, which can be difficult to differentiate from pneumonia in a patient with pulmonary shadowing and fever. Alveolar haemorrhage and organizing pneumonitis are more rarely seen complications of SLE. Treatment is with high-dose steroids or immunosuppression (e.g. cyclophosphamide). Pulmonary embolism (in the presence of the lupus 'anticoagulant') should always be considered as an alternative diagnosis for pulmonary shadowing, haemoptysis or pleurisy in a patient with SLE.

The respiratory muscles may be affected by a myopathy, which is most apparent when the diaphragm is affected; patients present with breathlessness and elevation of both hemi-diaphragms on the CXR. Immunosuppression with cyclophosphamide is preferable to high-dose steroids in view of the risk of further muscle wasting with the latter.

Systemic sclerosis

FA in systemic sclerosis is considered under the topic 'Diffuse parenchymal lung disease'. Pulmonary hypertension presents with breathlessness, signs of right ventricular hypertrophy, a normal CXR and impaired carbon monoxide transfer factor with well-preserved lung volumes. Intravenous prostacyclin infusion is beneficial in selected patients. Aspiration pneumonia is a complication of reduced oesophageal motility and, very rarely, cutaneous restriction of the expansion of the ribcage may occur.

Dermatomyositis/ polymyositis

These syndromes may be non-metastatic manifestations of a bronchial carcinoma. Respiratory complications such as fibrosing alveolitis and respiratory myopathy in these diseases are discussed under the topics 'Diffuse parenchymal lung diseases' and 'Neuromuscular disorders', respectively. Aspiration pneumonia may be seen when the oesophagus is affected.

Mixed connective

Mixed connective tissue disease can be associated with FA, pleural effusion, pulmonary hypertension, pulmonary embolism, and aspiration pneumonia.

Sjogren's syndrome

Pleural effusion, FA, lymphocytic pneumonitis and obliterative bronchiolitis have all been described as rare complications of Sjogren's syndrome.

Ankylosing spondylitis

Apical pulmonary fibrosis is seen in ankylosing spondylitis, which may cavitate. Fibrosing alveolitis is also seen, and pleural effusions have been reported. Restriction of ribcage expansion secondary to ankylosis is discussed under the topic 'Skeletal disorders'.

Further reading

Franck ST, Weg JG, Harkleroad LE, Fitch RF. Pulmonary dysfunction in rheumatoid disease. *Chest*, 1973; **63:** 27–34.

Vergnenegre A, Pugnere N, Antonin MT, Arnaud M, Melloni B, Treves B, Bonnaud F. Airway obstruction and rheumatoid arthritis. *European Respiratory Journal*, 1997; **10:** 1072–1078.

Pulmonary complications of systemic disease. In: Murray JF, ed. *Lung Biology in Health and Disease*, vol 59. Marcel Dekker, New York, 1992.

Related topics of interest

SARCOIDOSIS

Sarcoidosis is a multisystem disorder most commonly affecting the respiratory system, skin and eyes. It usually presents between the ages of 20 and 40 and is more common, more acute, and more severe in coloured races and is seen slightly more frequently in women.

Aetiology

Studies of sarcoidosis in nurses and contact tracing studies in the Isle of Man suggest person-to-person transmission or exposure to a common environmental agent. Various metal dusts, for example beryllium and organic antigens, can cause diseases with some similarities. There is little evidence otherwise that sarcoidosis is due to unrecognized environmental exposure.

The similarity of the disease to tuberculosis has suggested a mycobacterial origin. One study grew cell-wall-deficient forms of mycobacteria from blood of patients with active sarcoid, but the results of studies using PCR to detect mycobacterial DNA have been inconclusive.

Genetic factors are likely as familial clusters occur and it is more common in mono- than dizygotic twins. Genetic differences may influence T-cell function or antigen presentation and recognition. There is association with HLA-A1 and B8 (especially in those with erythema nodosum, acute arthritis or uveitis), and DR3.

It is likely that there are three events, exposure to antigen, acquired cellular immunity to antigen, and effector cells promoting a non-specific inflammatory response. The hallmark of the disease is the formation of non-caseating granulomata which can progress to fibrosis.

Clinical features

Sarcoidosis is often multisystem although it can apparently just involve one system. Extrapulmonary manifestations are as follows:

- Eyes (25%): see the topic 'Clinical examination'.
- Skin (25%): see the topic 'Clinical examination'.
- Nervous system (5%): seventh nerve palsy, unusual combinations of neurological signs.
- Liver (40–70%): hepatic granulomata; clinically significant disease uncommon.
- Splenomegaly (12%).
- Renal (1%): nephrocalcinosis (hypercalciuria ± hypercalcaemia), interstitial nephritis.
- Heart (5–10%): conduction abnormalities, sudden death, cardio-myopathy.
- Lymphadenopathy (25%).
- Upper respiratory tract (6%): often associated with lupus pernio, bone cysts.

- Hypercalcaemia (10%).

Respiratory involvement is usual at some point and presents as:

- Asymptomatic, for example found on CXR, with or without disease elswhere.
- Acute illness with erythema nodosum, bilateral hilar lymphadenopathy, arthralgia (Lofgren's syndrome).
- Chronic progressive breathlessness and cough with pulmonary infiltration, fibrosis and endobronchial disease.
- Upper respiratory tract, for example nasal mucosa, larynx.

Investigations

Chest radiology is conventionally staged:

- *Stage 1*: bilateral hilar lymphadenopathy (BHL) (approximately 65% of cases).
- *Stage 2*: BHL and pulmonary infiltration (approximately 22%).
- *Stage 3*: Infiltration without BHL (approximately 13%).

The differential diagnosis of these CXR appearances is as follows:

- Hilar lymphadenopathy: lymphoma, cancer, TB, beryllium, enlarged pulmonary arteries.
- Hilar lymphadenopathy and infiltration: TB, lymphangitis carcinomatosa, pneumoconiosis, alveolar cell carcinoma.
- Diffuse infiltration: pneumoconiosis, FA, EAA, lymphangitis carcinomatosa.

The HRCT findings in sarcoidosis consist of peribronchovascular interstitial thickening and nodules, fibrosis and conglomerate masses. Mediastinal lymph node enlargement is usual.

Confirmation of the diagnosis by biopsy is strongly recommended (from the least invasive site), especially when treatment is being considered. Transbronchial biopsy shows non-caseating granulomata in up to 80% of cases. BAL will show a lymphocytic alveolitis with a predominence of CD4 cells – though this test is not done routinely.

Urea and electrolytes, liver function tests and calcium should be measured routinely. Serum angiotensin converting enzyme is of too poor sensitivity and specificity to be of diagnostic use. A polyclonal increase in gamma globulins is common and hypercalcaemia and hypercalciuria occur in up to 10%.

Minimum lung function tests are spirometry and diffusion capacity. Lung function tests may be normal (e.g. with bilateral hilar lymphadenopathy), or may show a restrictive pattern with reduced gas transfer if interstitial disease is present. The tuberculin test is negative in two-thirds of cases and a strongly positive test is unusual. The Kveim test (intradermal injection of a homogenate of spleen from a sarcoid patient) has fallen into disuse because of concerns over transmissable agents.

Diagnosis relies on a compatible clinical picture and the exclusion of other granulomatous conditions (e.g. TB, beryllium, EAA, lymphoma, etc).

Management

Most patients should initially be observed because there is potential for improvement. Steroids are indicated in ocular, neurological, cardiac, and symptomatic pulmonary disease, and hypercalcaemia. A recent British Thoracic Society (BTS) study showed that patients with persistent CXR shadowing had a better long-term outcome if treated with steroids.

Steroids are the first line of therapy. There is no standard protocol but most clinicians start at about 40 mg daily with a reducing course over the next 6–12 months. Methotrexate is probably the second-line drug of choice at 10–15 mg/week, and should be considered in patients with a poor steroid response, or in those who recurrently relapse if steroids are reduced. Chloroquine is of benefit in skin sarcoid. Inhaled steroids have shown little convincing benefit.

Outcome

Remission without treatment occurs in roughly 60–80% of Stage 1 (especially Lofgren's syndrome), 50–60% in Stage 2, and less than 30% in Stage 3. About 50% have at least a mild degree of permanent dysfunction and this risk is higher in the coloured population, those without erythema nodosum, those aged over 40 years at onset, and those with widespread disease.

Serum ACE levels, Gallium scanning and lymphocyte count at BAL are not helpful in predicting disease progression. Vital capacity and gas transfer are the best lung function indices of assessment.

Further reading

Gibson GJ, Prescott RJ, Muers M *et al*. British Thoracic Society sarcoidosis study: effects of long term corticosteroid treatment. *Thorax*, 1996; **51:** 238–247.

Gottleib JE, Israel HI, Steiner RM, Triolo J, Patrick H. Outcome in sarcoidosis. The relationship of relapse to corticosteroid therapy. *Chest*, 1997; **111:** 623–631.

Related topics of interest

SKELETAL DISORDERS

Rib and sternal abnormalities

Multiple rib fractures may result in a flail segment. Intubation and ventilation may be necessary.

Pectus excavatum or carinatum and most congenital deformities of the ribs are usually only of cosmetic importance, only rarely interfering with the respiratory function of the ribcage.

Kyphosis

Kyphosis also has surprisingly little effect on respiration. Occasionally a severe kyphosis, usually following tuberculosis of one or more thoracic vertebrae in childhood, can lead to ventilatory failure.

Scoliosis

Scoliosis is a rotational deformity. Expansion of the lungs is restricted if the thoracic spine is involved, either as the primary site or in compensation for a lumbar curve. Scoliosis developing before the age of 5 years is particularly likely to cause respiratory problems later in life, possibly because impaired expansion of the lungs in infancy leads to sub-normal alveolar growth.

1. Congenital. Congenital absence of a hemivertebra or fusion of adjacent hemivertebrae inevitably leads to spinal curvature which becomes more marked as the normal side of the spine grows.

2. Idiopathic. Idiopathic scoliosis can first arise in infancy or adolescence. It is more common in females and with curvature convex to the left.

3. Paralytic. Weakness of the paraspinal muscles, for example after poliomyelitis or in spinal muscular atrophy, leads to scoliosis.

Surgery may be undertaken to stabilize the spine and prevent progression of the curvature, but in itself does not lead to significant improvement in respiratory function. Bracing is now seldom used. Non-invasive ventilation may be necessary if the patient develops hypercapnic respiratory failure, or symptomatic nocturnal hypoventilation.

Ankylosing spondylitis

Fusion of the costo-vertebral joints in ankylosing spondylitis can immobilize the ribcage, but diaphragmatic function is well preserved and respiratory failure is unusual in this condition.

Thoracoplasty

The operation of thoracoplasty was commonly performed for pulmonary tuberculosis in the 1950s, and is occasionally still performed for empyema. Removal of the ribs causes a small hemithorax, but also destabilizes the spine and produces a mild to moderate scoliosis. Associated pleural and pulmonary scarring from tuberculosis is usual. Hypercapnic respiratory failure is a common late complication, which usually responds well to non-invasive nocturnal assisted ventilation.

Lung function tests Spirometry is the simplest way to assess the extent to which the skeletal abnormality is restricting expansion of the lungs, and to monitor progression. Ventilatory failure is unlikely to develop in patients with a vital capacity of 2l or more. Lung volumes are also low, but the RV may be reduced less than TLC: in addition to being difficult to expand, the ribcage may resist compression below FRC by the expiratory muscles. Since the lungs are small, TLCO is also low, but the density of blood in the lungs is such that the KCO is high – the classical picture of extra-pulmonary restriction.

Further reading

Shneerson J. *Disorders of Ventilation.* Oxford: Blackwell, 1988.

Related topics of interest

Lung function tests (p. 102)
Neuromuscular disorders (p. 111)
Non-invasive ventilation (p. 114)

SLEEP APNOEA

Sleep apnoea, as its name suggests, involves cessation of breathing during sleep. Hypoventilation, as opposed to complete apnoea, produces much the same effects, but 'sleep apnoea/hypopnoea syndrome' is too cumbersome a term. Most sleep apnoea is the result of obstruction of the upper airway, and so obstructive sleep apnoea (OSA) is a convenient abbreviation. Estimates of the prevalence of OSA vary, depending partly upon the degree of obesity of the population but also on the diagnostic techniques and definition used; about 1–5% of the population of the UK are affected.

Aetiology

- Obesity of the neck – as indicated by a collar size greater than 16.5 inches.
- Tonsillar enlargement is the commonest cause of OSA in children, but may also cause the syndrome in adults.
- Hypothyroidism, acromegaly and amyloidosis are all associated with macroglossia which can obstruct the upper airway.
- Retrognathia may also contribute to upper airway narrowing.

Clinical features

Patients with OSA always snore, and usually do so irrespective of the position in which they sleep. A partner may report that the snoring is interrupted by apnoeic episodes, terminated by a gasp or snort. Sometimes the patient may awake with the sensation of choking.

Sleep is restless and interrupted, with the result that it is unrefreshing. Excessive sleepiness during the daytime leads to the patient falling asleep easily against their will, for example during meals or conversation. Driving accidents may occur, particularly during monotonous journeys on motorways. The Epworth Sleepiness Score can be used to quantify daytime sleepiness.

On examination, the size of the neck, tongue, tonsils and pharynx should be assessed. The degree of overbite is a guide to the presence of retrognathia. Cyanosis and right heart failure are features of severe OSA.

Investigations

Overnight oximetry charateristically shows dips in oxygen saturation of more than 4%, occurring at a rate of 15 or more per hour. Video recording is useful to confirm that these dips are indeed the result of obstructive apnoeas in equivocal cases. Polysomnography is the gold standard, with monitoring of airflow, chest wall motion and electroencephalography to allow staging of sleep. Thyroid function tests should be measured in all obese subjects.

Treatment

Weight loss, cessation of smoking, and avoidance of alcohol in the evening are advisable, but seldom effective in isolation. CPAP applied through a nasal mask is the treatment of choice for most patients. A chin strap or full face mask are sometimes required if the patient's mouth falls open during sleep.

Tonsillectomy is indicated if large tonsils are encroaching on the airway. The operation of uvulopalatopharyngoplasty is more effective for snoring than for OSA, but can be tried if CPAP cannot be tolerated. Some surgeons advocate nasendoscopy under sedation to detect the site of pharyngeal collapse prior to uvulopalatoplasty.

Mandibular advancement splints are available, but their place is still under evaluation. Surgical advancement of the mandible is also in its infancy. Tracheostomy was the only treatment before the introduction of CPAP, but is now very rarely used.

Further reading

Stradling JR. *Handbook of Sleep-related Breathing Disorders*. Oxford: Oxford University Press, 1993.

Related topics of interest

Non-invasive ventilation (p. 114)
Upper airway obstruction (p. 161)

THORACIC SURGICAL PROCEDURES

Rigid bronchoscopy

The use of the rigid metal bronchoscope, under general anaesthetic (GA), has several advantages. Ventilation is controlled allowing a more stable view of lesions in the bronchial tree. The larger tube diameter allows bigger biopsies than can be taken at fibreoptic bronchoscopy, and control of bleeding is much easier.

A disadvantage of rigid bronchoscopy is the requirement for GA, incurring morbidity and expense. The lack of flexibility makes viewing and taking biopsies from the upper lobes more difficult, though right-angled biopsy instruments overcome this to some extent, and if necessary a fibrescope can also be passed down the rigid scope.

Some procedures almost always need rigid bronchoscopy, for example extraction of foreign bodies, laser therapy, etc.

Thoracoscopy

A thoracoscope is a rigid metal instrument which, with a light source, is inserted into the pleural space through a 1–2 cm incision in the mid-axillary line under local or general anaesthetic. Under GA, a double lumen endotracheal tube (ETT) can be used to ventilate one lung allowing good exposure of the pleural cavity on the other side.

Simple thoracoscopy with this instrument has been used by surgeons world-wide, and regularly by physicians in Europe, for nearly a century, to obtain diagnostic pleural biopsies under direct vision, and for therapy of pleural disorders such as insufflation of talc for pleurodesis.

The usual approach to the diagnosis of pleural effusion in the UK is to perform a closed pleural aspiration and biopsy, usually with an Abram's or Trucut needle. If these techniques yield negative results on adequate pleural tissue, thoracoscopy should be considered.

Thoracoscopy may be difficult in the presence of marked loculation. Open pleural biopsy may then be preferable through a 7–10 cm incision. Thoracoscopy is particularly helpful in mesothelioma, which can be difficult to diagnose at closed biopsy. In one study, closed biopsy had about 40% sensitivity for the diagnosis of mesothelioma compared with 98% for thoracoscopy. Thoracoscopy has approximately a 95% sensitivity generally in malignant pleural disease.

Mediastinoscopy

Mediastinoscopies are carried out under GA via a short incision in the suprasternal notch, through which a rigid scope is passed behind the pre-tracheal fascia to view mediastinal structures. The technique allows biopsy of glands, mainly in the superior mediastinum. Complications occur in approximately 1%, and include bleeding, infection and vocal cord palsy.

Assessment of the mediastinum is crucial in the pre-operative staging of lung cancer. A conventional approach is to pre-operatively biopsy mediastinal glands (usually via mediastinoscopy, occasionally via anterior mediastinotomy), if CT scanning shows glands greater than 1 cm in diameter.

Mediastinoscopy is also used to obtain histology in other mediastinal glandular disease, for example sarcoidosis, tuberculosis, lymphoma, if there are no other glands that are more easily accessible.

Open/thoracoscopic lung biopsy

1. Diffuse parenchymal lung disease. TBB via the fibrescope is the procedure of choice for bronchocentric conditions such as sarcoidosis or cancer. If TBB is negative (and there is no other accessible biopsy site), or there is a condition in which TBB is unlikely to make a diagnosis (e.g. CFA or some rare DPLDs), then a surgical biopsy is required if histology is needed.

Conventional open lung biopsy carried out through a 7–10 cm incision in the right submammary fold has an operative mortality of under 1% and gives an accurate diagnosis in over 90%.

Video-assisted thoracoscopic surgical lung biopsy (VATS) is now the procedure of choice; initial comparisons with conventional open lung biopsy show a longer operating time but fewer complications and shorter hospital stays (in one study 5 days for VATS compared with 12 days for open lung biopsy).

Ventilator-dependent patients may still require an open lung biopsy but care should be taken in such patients as the procedure may rarely change outcome in this situation.

2. Lung nodules/masses. Most central and peripheral lung masses are diagnosable with a combination of clinical evaluation, non-invasive imaging and non-surgical diagnostic tools, such as fibreoptic bronchoscopy or percutaneous needle biopsy. In a small number of cases it is necessary to perform exploratory thoracotomy which can proceed to resection if necessary.

The VATS procedure has also been developed for biopsy of a solitary peripheral nodule – in one study showing 100% sensitivity and specificity in the diagnosis of both benign and malignant lesions. However, the major technical problem with this technique, and cause of failure in routine practice, is intraoperative localization of small nodules.

Further reading

Hetzel MR. *Minimally Invasive Techniques in Thoracic Medicine and Surgery*. London: Chapman and Hall, 1995.

Related topics of interest

Biopsy techniques (p. 22)
Fibre-optic bronchoscopy (p. 79)
Lung cancer (p. 97)

TRANSPLANTATION

Transplantation has transformed the management of several lung diseases which affect younger people. Combined heart–lung transplantation is used for conditions such as Eisenmenger syndrome or primary pulmonary hypertension. Lung transplantation with preservation of the recipient's own heart is appropriate for many patients with lung disease, since cardiac function will recover post-operatively, even in the presence of cor pulmonale. Single lung transplantation is appropriate for diseases such as FA, where immunosuppression poses no risk from the diseased lung which is left in place. Double lung (or heart–lung) transplantation is necessary in suppurative lung diseases such as bronchiectasis and CF.

Indications

CF, bronchiectasis, DPLDs and emphysema are the main indications for transplantation. Occasionally, patients with acute illnesses such as ARDS have been transplanted.

Transplantation should be considered in severe lung disease that is unresponsive to optimal medical therapy. Most patients in this category will have an FEV_1 of less than 30% and cor pulmonale, although it is appropriate to assess patients well above this level if their lung function is declining rapidly, for example in an adolescent with CF and in patients with FA after failure of first-line medical therapy. Patients over the age of 60 years are unlikely to be accepted for transplantation.

Contra-indications

The requirement for immunosuppression after transplantation means that active infection in extra-pulmonary sites is a contra-indication. Renal impairment will preclude the use of cyclosporin and is therefore a contra-indication. Patients who are malnourished do badly post-operatively. Poor rehabilitation potential, either because of physical illness or psychosocial problems is a contra-indication, as is current smoking.

Complications

1. Early. Within 1 month of transplantation, patients may experience acute rejection or graft-versus-host disease, whilst immunosuppresion predisposes to infections. During this period patients will be under the supervision of the surgical centre, with close monitoring of lung function and the radiographic appearances of the transplanted lung. Trans-bronchial biopsy and/or BAL may be necessary.

2. Late. Obliterative bronchiolitis is the most problematic late complication of transplantation, which may require intensification of immunosuppresive therapy or re-transplantation. Frequent monitoring of FEV_1 is mandatory and, if there is a decline, it may be necessary to perform a trans-bronchial biopsy. HRCT scanning may show changes suggestive of obliterative bronchiolitis.

Recurrence of the underlying disease in the transplanted lung has been described for a number of different diseases. Lymphoma may occur as a consequence of immunosuppression. Cyclosporin frequently causes renal damage.

Outcome The 1-year survival following transplantation is steadily improving, the current figures being in the region of 60–70%.

Further reading

International guidelines for the selection of lung transplant candidates. *American Journal of Respiratory Critical Care Medicine*, 1998; **158:** 335–339.

Related topics of interest

Bronchiectasis (p. 28)
Cystic fibrosis (p. 52)
Diffuse parenchymal lung disease (p. 59)
Emphysema (p. 69)
Pulmonary hypertension (p. 139)

UNUSUAL RESPIRATORY INFECTIONS

The number of organisms which may infect the lungs is extremely large, and many of the commoner ones are discussed under topics elsewhere in this book. Many of the remainder are so rare, or restricted to such a small geographical area, that they do not warrant detailed coverage in a text such as this. Some infections which may occasionally be encountered are described below.

Protozoa

Echinococcus granulosus is contracted from sheep and causes hydatid cysts in the lungs. The characteristic CXR appearances are of an abscess with an air fluid level, on the surface of which daughter cysts may be seen floating – sometimes referred to as the 'waterlily' sign. The cysts may rupture into pleura, causing an empyema, or into a bronchus leading to wheeze and production of blood-stained sputum. Eosinophilia is almost invariable. Diagnosis is made on the basis of serology or microsocopy of sputum or pleural fluid. Treatment is with albendazole.

Fungi

Cryptococcus neoformans is contracted from pigeons, with an acute illness characterized by cough, sputum, fever, malaise and weight loss. The illness is usually self-limiting, but large cryptococcomas can form and even cavitate. Amphotericin and 5-fluorocytosine are used in severe disease.

Histoplasma capsulatum is contracted from bird and bat droppings. It causes an acute illness with cough, fever, malaise, chest pain, dyspnoea. On the CXR there are bilateral infiltrates with mediastinal adenopathy. Chronic (often disseminated) disease occurs subsequently in about 10% of cases. Cavitation and calcification of the pulmonary lesions may occur. The diagnosis is made on sputum and blood cultures, biopsy specimens or serology. Amphotericin is used in severe acute and all chronic cases.

Bacteria

Nocardia asteroides causes consolidation or a more discrete mass, sometimes with cavitation, in patients with underlying lung disease or impaired immunity. Trimethoprim-sulphamethoxazole therapy is needed for at least 6 weeks. Imipenem, cefotaxime, amikacin and minocycline are alternatives.

Actinomyces israeli causes cough, sputum, haemoptysis, chest pain and weight loss. The CXR appearances may show cavitating upper zone shadowing or a more discrete mass. Pleural spread leads to an empyema, and erosion into bony structures and skin is characteristic. Most cases resolve with penicillin administered for several weeks.

Further reading

Jerray M, Benzarti M, Garrouche A *et al*. Hydatid disease of the lungs: a survey of 386 cases. *American Review of Respiratory Disease,* 1992; **146:** 185–189.

Kinnear WJM, Macfarlane JT. A survey of thoracic actinomycosis. *Respiratory Medicine,* 1990; **84:** 57–59.

Menendez R, Cordero PJ, Santos M, et al. Pulmonary infection with Nocardia species: a report on 10 cases and review. *European Respiratory Journal,* 1997; **10:** 1542–1546.

Related topics of interest

UPPER AIRWAY OBSTRUCTION

The upper airway can be defined as the trachea, larynx, oropharynx and nasopharynx, and is mainly the domain of ear, nose and throat (ENT) surgeons. However, several disorders of this region are important for respiratory physicians, mainly because of their presentation with breathlessness. Obstruction of the upper airway during sleep is dealt with in the topic 'Sleep apnoea'.

Aetiology

Acute obstruction of the upper airway can result from inhalation of a foreign body which lodges in the larynx, epiglottis or angio-oedema. A more insidious onset is seen with tumours of the trachea or larynx.

Benign or malignant thyroid swellings may compress the trachea. Retro-sternal extension is common in benign goitres. Because of the slow progression of the airway narrowing the patient may become used to the sensation of breathlessness and not realize the extent of their limited exercise tolerance.

Vocal cord paralysis is usually unilateral and presents with hoarseness rather than breathlessness. A left vocal cord palsy is an important indicator of mediastinal glandular invasion by a carcinoma. Bilateral paralysis of the cords can cause upper airway obstruction when the cords are immobilized in the adducted position. Laryngeal spasm produces upper airway wheeze which may be difficult to distinguish from asthma; it is associated with anxiety and hyperventilation.

Tracheal stenosis is a late complication of prolonged endo-tracheal intubation. Inflammatory conditions which may obstruct the upper airway include Wegener's granulomatosis (sub-glottic stenosis), sarcoidosis and relapsing polychondritis.

Clinical features

A careful history will usually distinguish these conditions from asthma, but misdiagnosis is common. Upper airway obstruction above the level of the suprasternal notch produces breathlessness which is worse when breathing in. The breathlessness of upper airway obstruction is more constant than that of asthma, with little variation within and between days or with bronchodilator treatment (although systemic steroids may reduce the size of a tumour obstructing the trachea and hence increase flow).

The cardinal sign of upper airway obstruction is stridor, this being noisy breathing particularly during inspiration, audible at the mouth without the aid of a stethoscope.

Investigations

A low but fairly constant peak flow should suggest the possibility of upper airway obstruction. The flow-volume loop is characteristic, with a flat plateau when flow is constant and does not vary with lung volume: this may be seen in both inspiration and expiration if the obstruction is fixed, or only on inspiration with a less rigid lesion above the level of the suprasternal notch, or only on expiration if it is below this point. Direct visualization using a rigid or fibre-optic endoscope and CT scanning are the investigations of choice.

Management

The method by which upper airway obstruction is relieved will depend on the aetiology of the obstruction, but may involve steroids, surgery, radiotherapy, laser therapy or stenting. Temporary relief can be obtained by inhalation of 'Heliox', a mixture of 80% helium and 20% oxygen – the density of this gas is much less than air, and the respiratory work involved in getting it through a narrow orifice is consequently much less.

Further reading

Miller MR, Pincock AC, Oates GD *et al*. Upper airway obstruction due to goitre: detection, prevalence and results of surgical mangement. *Quarterly Journal of Medicine*, 1990; **74:** 177–188.

Related topics of interest

VASCULITIS

The pulmonary vasculitic diseases include a range of conditions such as Wegener's granulomatosis and Churg Strauss syndrome with many overlapping features. Probably the best approach to classification of vasculitis is based on the size of vessels affected. Table 1 shows the main classes of vasculitis.

Table 1. The main classes of vasculitis

Vasculitis	Size of vessel	Pulmonary involvement
Takayasu's vasculitis	Major arteries	Rare
Giant cell arteritis	Large and medium arteries	Rare
Polyarteritis nodosa	Small and medium arteries	Rare
Microscopic polyangiitis	Small arteries	Uncommon
Churg Strauss syndrome	Small arteries + extra vascular granulomas	Common
Wegener's granulomatosis	Small arteries + extra vascular granulomas	Common

Churg Strauss syndrome

Churg Strauss syndrome is characterized by the combination of asthma, allergic rhinitis and peripheral eosinophilia. Essentially, any organ system can be affected and the features of this disease are therefore very variable. In most patients the pulmonary features and peripheral eosinophilia develop prior to other systemic involvement.

1. Clinical features. The clinical features of Churg Strauss syndrome depend upon the organ systems involved. Asthma is the most frequent presenting feature, often pre-dating other systemic involvement by several years. Asthma may be severe and require long-term steroid treatment. Allergic rhinitis also occurs at an early stage in the disease process. At a later stage, dermatological involvement is common: the most frequent abnormalities are a vasculitic rash, subcutaneous nodules and palpable purpura. Cardio-vascular disease is an important cause of long-term complications: acute pericarditis occurs in approximately one-third of patients; constrictive pericarditis and left ventricular impairment are also relatively common. Renal disease occurs less frequently than in other vascular disease (e.g. Wegener's granulomatosis) but glomerulonephritis does occur. Peripheral nerve involvement (most frequently mononeuritis multiplex) is common in late disease. Musculo-skeletal involvement can produce myalgia and polyarthritis. Finally, an eosinophilic gastroenteritis characterized by diarrhoea and abdominal pain also occurs.

2. Investigations. There is no specific laboratory investigation which enables a firm diagnosis of Churg Strauss syndrome to be made. Characteristic abnormalities on blood tests include striking peripheral eosinophilia ($>5 \times 10^9$ l), high ESR, normochromic normocytic anaemia and a positive pANCA titre (qv). The CXR during the acute stage shows transient infiltrates which may occur in any distribution. Both the radiological features and the peripheral eosinophilia are sensitive to steroid treatment. Small pleural effusions also frequently occur. HRCT shows no specific features of Churg Strauss syndrome. Lung function tests show features compatible with asthma.

The clinical diagnosis of Churg Strauss syndrome is supported by biopsy changes of an eosinophilic vasculitis present particularly in small arteries and veins: these features may be seen in a range of tissues, for example open lung biopsy or muscle biopsy. The American College of Rheumatology require four or more of the following criteria for the diagnosis of Churg Strauss syndrome:

- Asthma.
- Eosinophilia (>10 %).
- Transient pulmonary infiltrates.
- Paranasal sinus disease.
- Neuropathy.
- Biopsy changes showing eosinophilic vasculitis.

3. Management. Churg Strauss syndrome usually responds to high-dose prednisolone. Other immunosuppressive agents (cyclophosphamide, azathiaprine) may be required in severe disease.

4. Outcome. In general the prognosis is reasonably good unless multi-system involvement is present.

Wegener's granulomatosis

Wegener's granulomatosis is a systemic vasculitis affecting small- or medium-sized vessels. The spectrum of disease seen by respiratory physicians may be different from that seen by renal physicians: some patients having predominantly pulmonary rather than renal involvement and vice versa. Associated features of Wegener's granulomatosis are:

- Glomerulonephritis.
- Rash.
- Uveitis.
- Myositis.
- Mononeuritis multiplex.
- Myocarditis.
- Pericarditis.

1. Pulmonary manifestations. Wegener's granulomatosis presents with either upper or lower airway involvement, or both. Features of nasal disease include a bloody nasal discharge, nasal ulceration, rhinorrhea and sinusitis. Lower respiratory tract involvement usually presents with cough, haemoptysis, pleuritic chest pain and breathlessness. Upper airway disease may also present with stridor. There are usually associated systemic symptoms.

2. *Investigations.* A range of radiological abnormalities may be present on the CXR. Classically, cavitating nodules are observed: these may be several centimetres in diameter. Diffuse alveolar shadowing may also be present, particularly in the presence of pulmonary haemorrhage. Less common abnormalities include pleural effusions and hilar lymphadenopathy. The cavitating nature of pulmonary nodules is often well demonstrated on CT scanning. The demonstration of a classic vasculitis on either skin, nasal, renal or pulmonary biopsy is helpful in establishing the diagnosis.

Wegener's granulomatosis is often associated with a normochromic normocytic anaemia, elevated ESR, leucocytosis, and thrombocytosis. In patients with renal disease, renal impairment and an active urinary sediment are usual. Most patients with Wegener's granulomatosis have positive ANCA. ANCA may be either c-ANCA (characterized by autoantibodies against serum proteinase 3, the c standing for cytoplasmic pattern) or p-ANCA (antibodies against myeloperoxidase, the p indicating a perinuclear pattern of staining). Positive c-ANCA antibodies are found in almost all patients with Wegener's granulomatosis but are not specific for the disease, being also found in other vasculitides such as microscopic polyangiitis. In contrast, p-ANCA antibodies (particularly if present at low titre) are seen in a wide variety of other systemic inflammatory diseases and acute infections and are hence not diagnostic.

Patients with upper airway disease may have evidence of upper airway obstruction on flow volume loops. Pulmonary haemorrhage may produce an increased carbon monoxide transfer factor.

3. *Management and outcome.* Untreated Wegener's granulomatosis has a poor prognosis, with patients dying of progressive renal failure or pulmonary complications. Treatment is with immunosuppressive therapy and renal replacement therapy if indicated. Cyclophosphamide induces remission in up to 75% of patients; however, half of these will suffer relapse at some stage.

Further reading

Burns A. Pulmonary vasculitis. *Thorax*, 1998; **53:** 220–227.

Related topic of interest

Pulmonary eosinophilia (p. 137)

INDEX

Trauma, 1, 129
Tuberculosis, 1, 40, 42, 49, 65, 72, 74, 79, 90, 105–109, 150

Ulcerative colitis, 64
Ultrasound, 89

Upper airway obstruction, 161–162

Vasculitis, 28, 163–164
Ventilation/perfusion scanning, 88, 135

Wegener's granulomatosis, 41, 42, 164